Contents

Introduction
A Stevens, J Raftery

Child and Adolescent Mental Health
SA Wallace, JM Crown, M Berger, AD Cox

Foreword

Everyone involved in the purchasing, planning and prioritization of health care needs accurate, comprehensive and well-packaged information to answer at least four crucial questions. With what population or patients are we concerned? What services are provided? What is the evidence of the effectiveness of services? What is the optimum set of services? In other words: What is the need and how can it be best met?

These questions are answered in part by epidemiological literature and in part by the products of the evidence-based health care movement. The *Health Care Needs Assessment* series neatly combines these two elements and offers a perspective across an entire disease or service area. A purchaser or practitioner reading one of these chapters is rapidly brought up-to-speed with the whole spectrum of care.

Many positive comments, including evidence supplied to the House of Commons' Health Committee, have demonstrated the value and importance of the first series. The additional topics in the second series extend the range of information available covering both areas where the assessment of need and effectiveness of services has long been discussed, such as aspects of gynaecology and low back pain, and ones in which there has been less interest, such as dermatology. The new series will be welcomed by purchasers of health care in the United Kingdom but it should also be of value to all those concerned with assessing and meeting health care needs, from central government to individual practitioners.

Graham Winyard
Medical Director, NHS Executive
September 1996

Preface

contributing authors

This book forms part of the second series of health care needs assessment reviews. The first series, published in 1994, comprises reviews of 20 diseases, interventions or services selected for their importance to purchasers of health care. Importance is defined in terms of burden of disease (mortality, morbidity and cost), the likely scope for changing patterns of purchasing and the wish to see a wide range of topics to test the method used for needs assessment. The first series also includes an introductory chapter, explaining the background to needs assessment and a conclusive chapter, bringing together the main findings of the disease reviews.

The eight reports have been chosen, using the same importance criteria to increase the coverage of all health service activity. There has been a small change in emphasis, away from disease groups (strictly *Breast Cancer* only), to services and in some cases entire specialties (*Dermatology* and *Gynaecology*). The change has been partly to maintain coverage of substantial areas in each report (where otherwise a relatively small disease group would now require an individual chapter) and also to reflect the wishes of the users for the topic areas to be consistent with the scope of purchasing plans if at all possible.

As before the authors have been selected on the basis of academic expertise and each chapter is the work of individual authors. The reviews do not necessarily reflect the views of the National Health Service Executive that sponsored the project, nor indeed the current professional consensus. Each review should be in no way regarded as setting norms; rather it should be used as a valuable source of evidence and arguments on which purchasing authorities may base their decisions.

There have been other changes since the first series which have influenced the range of reviews and the content of individual reviews. First districts have merged and a population base of 250 000 is no longer the norm. Denominators are now expressed as per 100 000, or per million population. Second the term purchasers no longer strictly means just district health authorities. Some small steps have therefore been taken in the direction of making the material relevant to primary care purchasing. This is particularly so in the *Low Back Pain* review, in which the focus is on the presenting symptom as in general practice rather than on a confirmed diagnosis following secondary care. Third the science of systematic reviews and meta-analyses has developed remarkably since the production of the first series. While this important development has been of great use to purchasers, the role of the needs assessment in covering entire disease and service areas remains unique. Both objectives of providing baseline information for purchasers to assist with the knowledge-base of all the processes around purchasing and designing a method for needs assessment have largely been vindicated by comments received on the first series and the demand for a second series.

The editors wish to acknowledge the contribution of those who helped with the origination of the project: Graham Winyard, Mike Dunning, Deirdre Cunningham and Azim Lakhani; and also members of the current Steering Group: Mark Charny, Anne Kauder and Graham Bickler; as well as those at Wessex who have enabled the project to run smoothly: Ros Liddiard, Pat Barrett and Melanie Corris.

Contributing authors

Berger, Dr M
Consultant Clinical Psychologist
Department of Clinical Psychology
Lanesborough Wing
St George's Hospital
Blackshaw Road
LONDON SW17 0QT

Cox, Professor AD
UMDS
Department of Adolescent Psychiatry and Psychology
Bloomfield Centre
Guy's Hospital
London Bridge
LONDON SE1 9RT

Crown, Dr JM
Director
South East Institute of Public Health
Broomhill House
David Salomon's Estate
Broomhill Road
TUNBRIDGE WELLS TN3 0XT

Wallace, Dr SA
Senior Registrar in Public Health Medicine
South East Institute of Public Health
Broomhill House
David Salomon's Estate
Broomhill Road
TUNBRIDGE WELLS TN3 0XT

Introduction

A Stevens, J Raftery

Needs assessment means different things according to who uses the term, when and where. Some of these uses are reviewed in this introduction. Our understanding of needs assessment stems from the wish to provide useful information for those involved in the priority setting and purchasing of health care.

We are concerned with population health care need and define it as 'the population's ability to benefit from health care'[1,2,3] as did Culyer 20 years ago.[4] Mention of health care is important because for the purposes of commissioning health services it is crucial that there be some benefit from the interventions that follow from the assessment of need. The benefit can be immediate or in the future, physical or psychological, personal or communal. The intervention can concern health promotion, diagnosis, or palliation as well as treatment. We argue that needs are worth assessing when something useful can be done about them. The two essential determinants of a population's ability to benefit are the:

- incidence and/or prevalence of a health problem
- effectiveness of the interventions available to deal with it.

These two components form the core of the protocol used in the chapters that follow.

Current service provision although not a determinant of need is also highly relevant if needs assessment is to have any value in action. We need to know how things stand before we can change them. The reliance of our approach on these three elements is shown in Figure 1. The effectiveness corner of the triangle includes *cost*-effectiveness because this allows us to consider the *relative* priority of different needs.

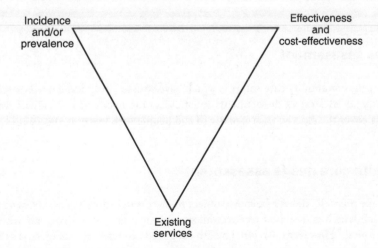

Figure 1: The elements of health care needs assessment.

We also distinguish need from demand (what people would be willing to pay for or might wish to use in a system of free health care) and from supply (what is actually provided).[1,2,3] This helps to classify health service interventions according to whether they reflect need, demand or supply (or some combination). It also highlights the need for caution in the use of information sources which often say more about supply (e.g. utilization rates) or demand (e.g. patient preference surveys) than they do about need. It also reminds health care commissioners of the importance of drawing together needs, supply and demand as shown in Figure 2. The central area of overlap is the optimum field for service provision, i.e. where need, supply and demand are congruent.

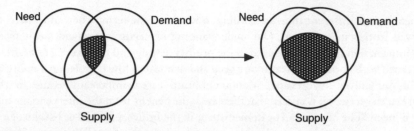

Figure 2: Drawing need, demand and supply together: the role of the purchasers of health care.

We also suggest three practical tools for health care needs assessment (see page xvi):

1 epidemiological
2 comparative
3 corporate.

Alternative approaches

There is a considerable range of alternative approaches to needs assessment depending on their purpose and context.

Social services assessment

In UK public policy the community care reforms which have stressed individual needs assessment for social care. Local authority social services departments must assess the needs of individuals for personal social services that mainly cover the elderly, the mentally ill and people with learning disabilities.[5]

Individual health care needs assessment

In health care too, the mentally ill have become subject to increased individual assessment through the care programme approach which is designed to cover all severely mentally ill individuals who are about to be discharged from hospital.[6] However individual health care needs assessment has existed as long as medicine and is the key feature of much of health care. The clinical focus regards need as the best that can be done for a patient in a particular setting. In primary care the establishment of routine health checks in the UK, especially for the over 75s, is an example of formalized individual needs assessment, which raised controversy in its imposition of mass individual needs assessment that includes people who are not necessarily in any need.[7,8]

Participatory priority setting

In the US needs assessment is often used as a term for participatory priority setting by organizations, which are usually public sector or voluntary rather than for profit. These involve three elements: defining the needs of organizations or groups, setting priorities and democratic involvement.[9] At state level the now famous Oregon approach to priority setting has much in common with needs assessment for health care commissioning in the UK but the explicit use of the participatory democratic element in the US was striking.[10] Even in the UK health policy since 1991 has attributed growing importance to the role of the public. This has been both in the form of central exhortation[11,12] and in local practice as many district health authorities have tried to involve the public in priority setting.[13] Public involvement has also occurred unintentionally through the media: a series of controversial cases, notably Child B who was denied a second NHS funded bone marrow transplant for leukaemia on the basis of the likely ineffectiveness of the treatment, have raised national debates.[14]

Primary care approaches

Other approaches, some imposed from above and some experimental from below are emerging from attempts to establish needs assessment in primary care. The routine assessment of the over 75s is an example of a top-down initiative and is unusual in requiring individual needs assessment by general practitioners of an entire age group.[7,8] Bottom-up experimental approaches tend to be based around data gathering through different means including for example rapid participatory appraisal, the analysis of routinely available small area statistics and the collation of practice-held information.[15,16] The analysis of small area statistics has a long tradition, including the use of Jarman indicators[17] and belongs to the comparative method of health care needs assessment – principally identifying a need for further analysis. Examining practice-held information including the audit of general practice case notes has had a growing role and is potentially much more relevant to population needs assessment than audit in secondary care. Because primary care case notes have a wide population coverage (90% of a practice population in three years) and each primary health care team has a relatively small population, it is possible for a primary health care team to expose practice population needs (given a knowledge of the effectiveness of interventions) through case note analysis. The development of computerized case notes in general practice could dramatically increase the scope for this approach.

Local surveys

In health authorities the use of local surveys has increased. These can cover multiple client groups and involve the collection of objective morbidity data. Local bespoke surveys of morbidity[18] can be supplemented by the interpretation of semi-routine data from national surveys such as the General Household Survey[19] and the OPCS Disability Survey.[20,21] Directors of Public Health annual health reports often include both local surveys and elements of such data. These can collect valuable information, although there is a risk that when local surveys are both limited to a selective range of client groups, and are centred around subjective information, they will give disproportionate importance to a selective range of interests.

Specialty-specific documents

Documents setting out the service requirements of client groups of an individual specialty are sometimes also treated as needs assessments. These often recommend the augmentation of services (within that specialty). Their validity as needs assessment documents depends on the explicitness and thoroughness of their research base.

Clinical effectiveness research

Finally, perhaps the most important contribution to needs assessment has been the major expansion of clinical effectiveness research in the UK and elsewhere. In the UK the Department of Health's research programme and especially its emphasis on 'health technology assessment' is a major attempt to evaluate the effectiveness of many health care interventions and therefore inform the health care needs which underlie them.[22,23]

In determining the differences between these various approaches to needs assessment it is helpful to ask the following questions:

1 **Is the principal concern with health or social services?** The effectiveness component of need for social services is often not recognized. The reason for this may be that there is seldom a clear-cut distinction between what works and what does not. More housing or more education is seldom seen as undesirable. In health care, by contrast, some interventions work spectacularly well but a point arises at which increased intervention *is* undesirable. Excessive medication or surgery may not only be of no benefit but can be harmful. It could be argued that in social care the potential open-endedness of benefit and therefore of spending makes it more important to assess the effectiveness of interventions and make a judgement of what the need is. The spectre of rationing in a politically charged context often deters such explicitness.

2 **Is the needs assessment about population or individuals?** Many approaches to needs assessment are necessarily concerned with individuals. Local authority social services programmes and primary care health checks focus on individuals. Traditional clinical decision making and also some purchasing decisions such as extra-contractual referrals concern individuals. The media focus is almost always on the individual. Although individual needs assessment can be seen as the opposite end of the spectrum from population based needs assessment the underlying logic is the same.

    The purchaser (population needs assessor) is concerned with meeting the aggregate needs of the population. For some client groups where individuals are either few or prominent in their health care costs, such as in the case of mentally disordered offenders they may well need to be individually counted or even individually assessed to provide the population picture.[24,25] Wing *et al.* consider the purchaser's population view and the individual clinical view of mental health need to be 'largely identical'.[26] In part they say this because individual needs can be aggregated but in part they recognize the importance of service effectiveness as integral to the need equation.

3 **Is there a clear context of allocating scarce resources?** Needs assessments that fail to acknowledge resource limitations are common but are of restricted value to health care commissioners. This can be a problem with individual clinical needs assessment, which can put great pressure on health budgets and squeeze the care available to patients with weak advocates. However clinicians work within an (often) implicit resource framework. Population health care needs assessment makes that framework explicit. Some population approaches also fail to acknowledge resource issues. This can be a problem with population surveys if they are neither set in the context of effectiveness, nor make it clear that they are

exploratory. It is also a difficulty with specialty-specific documents recommending levels of service within the specialty.[27] Examples abound as many specialties are anxious to protect or enhance the resources available to them.[28] This may be justified but they risk being little more than a group extension of an unbounded clinical decision making procedure.

4 **Is the needs assessment about priority setting within the context of a variety of competing needs or is it about advocacy for a single group or individual?** This is closely related to the resource context question. Specialty-specific documents, client group surveys and even policy directives which focus on single groups often represent advocacy rather than balanced contributions to priority setting. Surveys about, for example, the needs of a particular ethnic minority are of limited help in guiding purchasers unless seen in the context of equivalent surveys of other groups. Whether a policy directive is advocacy based or priority based depends on how it comes about. A set of recommendations based on lobbying will be much more prone to distorting resource use than one based on research. Arguably the Child B case moved from a priority setting to an advocacy framework when the debate moved from the health authority to the law courts.

5 **Is the needs assessment exploratory or definitive?** Some approaches to needs assessment are exploratory in that they highlight undefined or under-enumerated problems. This is particularly true of lifestyle surveys that estimate the size of risk groups such as alcohol abusers or teenage smokers. Surveys of the needs within specific client groups can also fall within this category but they differ from population surveys in that they often involve advocacy. If effectiveness of interventions has been determined prior to a population survey then this approach is compatible with epidemiological health care needs assessment.

6 **Is the determination of the most important needs expert or participatory?** The epidemiological approach to needs assessment is essentially an expert approach (with a population perspective). It seeks to be as objective as possible although no judgement of relative needs can be truly objective. Interpretation of data is partly subjective and the rules for decision making are inevitably value-laden. However the setting of priorities using an epidemiological and cost-effectiveness framework is markedly different from a process based on democratic consensus. Attempts to merge the two as in Oregon and in the local experience of many health authorities can have merit but the outcome will nearly always depend on the relative emphasis given to the provision of objective information and the extent to which participants can interpret them. As a general rule the expert approach to priority setting is more viable the further it is from the clinical decision making. At one extreme the World Health Organization's assessment of relative need operates by very clear cost-effectiveness rules.[29] At the other extreme the individual clinical decisions are rightly very open to patient views. District health authorities have to reconcile the two.

Underlying all of these questions is the further question: 'Who carries out the needs assessment and for what purpose?' Provided the assessment's aims and context are clearly stated and clearly understood there is a place for all of these approaches to needs assessment. Many can be subsumed within the approach used in this book in that they provide information about:

- numbers in a particular group, i.e. incidence and prevalence
- the effectiveness and cost-effectiveness of interventions
- the distribution of current services and their costs.

There is more information available on these elements of epidemiology-based needs assessment. Epidemiological studies contribute to the first point in the list above; effectiveness and outcomes research, i.e. evidence-based health care, to the second and assessments of current services to the third. The bringing together of the three themes in this book has been supported elsewhere at the extremes of individual and global needs assessments. For example Brewin's approach to measuring individual needs for mental health care identifies need as present when *both* function is impaired *and* when it is due to remedial cause.[30] Bobadilla *et al.*, in prescribing a minimum package for public health and clinical interventions for poor and middle income counties across all disease groups, identify both 'the size of the burden caused by a particular disease, injury and risk factor and the cost effectiveness of interventions to deal with it'.[29] Table 1 summarizes different approaches to health care needs assessment using the criteria discussed above.

Tools

In the first series of health care needs assessment we suggested three tools for needs assessment:

1 the epidemiological
2 comparative
3 corporate approaches.[2,3]

The definition of health care needs as the 'ability to benefit' implies an epidemiological approach. That is an assessment of how effective, for how many and, for the purposes of relative needs assessment, at what cost. However comparisons between localities (the comparative approach) and informed views of local service problems (the corporate approach) are important too.

The value of the 'comparative approach' is well demonstrated in the assessment of need for renal replacement therapy.[31] Increases in dialysis and transplantation in the UK closer to levels seen in better-provided European countries has been demonstrated over time to meet real needs. The need to change replacement levels from 20 per million in the 1960s, to 80 per million was suggested by both the comparative and epidemiological approach, i.e. of identifying incident end-stage renal failure and the effectiveness of renal replacement therapy. The comparative method does not however easily lead to cost-effectiveness considerations and is less successful in assessing which modality of renal replacement therapy is to be preferred; as the different balance between haemodialysis, peritoneal dialysis and transplantation rests on a variety of factors. The cost-effectiveness of different modalities is critical to priority setting. The comparative approach can however prompt key questions and therefore sets the priorities for more detailed analysis.

Almost every chapter of the first series of health care needs assessment expressed doubts about the extent and reliability of much of the routine data available for comparative analysis. The data on activity and prescribing, for example, would need to be linked to disease codes to represent faithfully true disease episodes. Disease registers such as those provided by the cancer registries can be invaluable and developments in information technology and unique patient numbers offer great scope for improved comparative analyses.

The 'corporate approach' involves the structured collection of the knowledge and views of informants on health care services and needs. Valuable information is often available from a wide range of parties, particularly including purchasing staff, provider clinical staff and general practitioners. Gillam points out that 'the intimate detailed knowledge of health professionals amassed over the years is often overlooked' and he particularly commends the insight of general practitioners, a suggestion well taken by many health authorities.[32] The corporate approach is essential if policies are to be sensitive to local circumstances. This approach might explore: first, a particularly prominent local need – such as the identification of severely mentally ill patients discharged from long-stay mental hospitals and lost to follow-up; second, consequences of local service considerations such as the balance between secondary and primary and local authority community care – as has been noted in the case of district nursing services;[33] third, where local needs differ from expectations based on national averages or typical expectations (due to local socioeconomic or environmental factors); and fourth, local popular concerns which may attach priorities to particular services

Table 1: Different approaches to health care needs assessment

Criterium	Health/social focus	Individual population based	Resource/scarcity clear	Competing needs/advocacy	Definitive/exploratory	Expert/participatory
Population health care needs	Health	Population	Yes	Competing	Definitive	Expert
Individual health care needs	Health	Individual	Sometimes	Either	Definitive	Expert
Social services assessments	Social	Individual	Sometimes	Competing	Both	Both
Participatory planning	Social	Population	Sometimes	Competing	Definitive	Participatory
Oregon-style planning	Health	Population	Yes	Competing	Definitive	Both
Primary health care checks	Health	Individual	No	Competing	Exploratory	Expert
Primary health care case note audit	Health	Individual	No	Competing	Both	Expert
Population surveys	Health	Population	No	Competing	Exploratory	Expert
Client group surveys	Health	Population	No	Advocacy	Exploratory	Both
Specialty recommendations	Health	Population	No	Advocacy	Definitive	Expert
Effectiveness reviews	Health	Population	Yes	Competing	Definitive	Expert

or institutions (effectiveness considerations being equal). The need for cottage hospitals as opposed to large primary care units or other modes of community service provision might be an example. Clearly the potential pitfalls of informal corporate assessment of need are bias and vested interest that could cloud an objective view of the evidence. Nevertheless corporate memory should not be ignored.

The 'epidemiological approach' has been described fully.[3] It is worth reiterating that the epidemiological approach goes wider than epidemiology. It includes reviews of incidence and prevalence and also evidence about the effectiveness and relative cost-effectiveness of interventions, which, for service planners is increasingly seen as a focal concern. The epidemiological approach to needs assessment has helped pioneer what is now a sea-change towards evidence-based health care purchasing.

Evidence-based health care requires some rating of the quality of evidence. The first series required contributors to assess the strength of recommendation as shown in Table 2 adapted from the US Task Force on preventive health care.[34] This is now a mainstay of evidence-based medicine and it is retained in the present series.

Table 2: Analysis of service efficacy

Strength of recommendation	
A	There is good evidence to support the use of the procedure
B	There is fair evidence to support the use of the procedure
C	There is poor evidence to support the use of the procedure
D	There is fair evidence to reject the use of the procedure
E	There is good evidence to support the rejection of the use of the procedure

Quality of evidence	
(I)	Evidence obtained from at least one properly randomized controlled trial
(II-2)	Evidence obtained from well-designed cohort or case controlled analytic studies, preferably from more than one centre or research group
(II-3)	Evidence obtained from multiple timed series with or without the intervention, or from dramatic results in uncontrolled experiments
(III)	Opinions of respected authorities based on clinical experience, descriptive studies or reports of expert committees
(IV)[a]	Evidence inadequate owing to problems of methodology, e.g. sample size, length or comprehensiveness of follow-up, or conflict in evidence

Table adapted from US Task Force on Preventive Health Care.
[a]The final quality of evidence (IV) was introduced by Williams *et al.* for the surgical interventions considered in the first series.[35]

The changing background

Health care needs assessment was thrown into the spotlight in 1989 by the National Health Service Review.[36] The review, by separating purchasers and providers, identified population health care purchasing and therefore health care needs assessment as a distinct task. Since the beginning of the 1990s however a variety of circumstances has changed including the activities and research encompassed by health care needs assessment.

District health authority changes

The nature of the purchaser of health care at district health authority has changed in several ways. First, district mergers have resulted in larger purchasing units. Second the amalgamation of district health authorities with family health services authorities has extended the scope of purchasing and encouraged a more integrated approach to primary and secondary care services. Third the abolition of regional health authorities has necessitated careful purchasing of specialist services (these were formerly purchased regionally). Fourth the relationship between purchasers and providers of health care is showing some signs of maturing, as it has become obvious that large monopsonists (dominant purchasers) and monopolists have to work fairly closely together. Fifth there has been increased involvement of general practitioners (see below). These changes make districts potentially more sophisticated assessors of health care needs – although in practice such sophistication has been slowed by the administrative upheaval caused by the changes.

Cost containment

The second critical background circumstance affecting health care needs assessment is the increasing recognition of the need for cost containment. Although costs have always been constrained by the NHS allocation, new pressures have resulted from a variety of sources.

- Increased patient expectations – some of which have been encouraged centrally – particularly those concerning waiting times.
- New technologies with either a high unit cost, e.g. new drugs such as Beta Interferon for multiple sclerosis and DNase for cystic fibrosis, or which widen the indications for treatment, e.g. new joint replacement prostheses which have a longer life-span and can be given to younger patients.[37,38]
- New pressures at the boundaries between day health and social care in the problems of community care, and more recently with the criminal justice system – in the case of mentally disordered offenders.[39]

In theory the logic of needs assessment allows the identification of over-met need – in the sense of relatively ineffective and expensive services – as easily as undermet needs. In practice the former is more difficult to identify and much more difficult to correct. This further focuses attention on a limited number of areas and especially on a limited number of the most important cost pressures such as Beta Interferon.

General practitioner fundholding and GPs in purchasing

The third major background change has been the growing relative importance of general practice fundholding as a purchasing entity. In 1991 GP fundholding covered only around 10% of the population. One of the more striking aspects of the NHS reforms has been the expansion of fundholding which now (1996) covers more than half the population of England and Wales.[40] The scope of standard fundholding has been extended to cover the bulk of elective surgery outpatient care (except maternity and emergencies), community nursing and various direct access services. Some 70 total purchasing pilots have been established where GPs take on the entire NHS allocation for their patients. Side by side with these experiments in budget delegation is a variety of schemes whereby GPs are consulted, or otherwise involved in the commissioning of services.

Health care needs assessment in this book was designed primarily with district health authorities in mind. This reflected the dominant status of health authorities as purchasers at the time and also the size of the populations they covered. A population perspective makes more sense the larger the population, not least because the expected numbers of cases and their treatments are more predictable in larger populations. This is an issue for locality purchasing in general[41] and has even been a problem for district health authority purchasing when it comes to tertiary services and the rarer secondary services. The average GP sees only one case of thyroid cancer every 25 years and only eight heart attacks every year.[42] General practitioner fundholders cover populations ranging from 7000 to around 30 000. The total purchasing pilots which cover populations up to 80 000 only slightly ameliorate this. For GPs needs assessment as defined in this series is most likely to be applicable at the level of consortia with a large population. But taken together with GP involvement in profiling the population through case note audit and other means, needs assessment in primary care offers fruitful possibilities.

Evidence-based health care

The fourth main background change is in the drive from the research community itself. The evidence-based medicine and knowledge-based purchasing movement has been partly driven by imperatives to cost containment against a background of increasing health care costs as technology advances and by the acknowledgement that not all health care is effective[22,43] and by the differences in cost-effectiveness. The result is that needs assessment and cost-effectiveness assessment have become very closely related.

Use of the health care needs assessment series

Evidence for the usefulness of the epidemiological approach has come from the results of a survey of directors of public health in the UK[45], a Department of Health focus group on the first series, the House of Commons Health Committee's[46] review of the process by which authorities set priorities, and a national survey of contracting.[47] Two contrasting themes arising from these sources emerge.

1 There is an increasing appetite in health authorities for reliable material which assists priority setting. Health care purchasers are increasingly establishing a knowledge base across the whole range of health care, even if change is most effectively carried through by being reasonably selective.
2 Contracts themselves are not (yet) disease-based – usually built up from specialties they lack a starting point from which needs assessment can play a part. Thus although needs assessment has a role in setting the perspective for contracting, the guarantee that detailed implementation will take place is lacking. In part this reflects staffing shortages and the competing claims of other foci for purchasing (mergers, extra contractual referrals, waiting list initiatives, efficiency drives etc.). In part early attempts to develop disease-specific foci were hampered by poor quality data on patient treatment and particularly costs. This will become less of a problem not just with the growth of health technology assessment to provide the evidence base but also with initiatives such as the National Steering Group on Costing which has led to the costing of health care resource groups (HRGs) in six specialties.[48,49]

These surveys and experience with the first and second series have confirmed the usefulness of the protocol for health care needs assessment. Its six main elements remain:

1 a statement of the problem (normally a disease or intervention)
2 identifying the relevant sub-categories

3   the incidence and prevalence of the condition
4   the nature and level of service provided
5   the effectiveness (including the cost–effectiveness) of the service or treatments
6   models of care.

In addition authors have considered appropriate outcome measures, targets, the routine information available and current research priorities.

To extend the coverage and to link health care needs assessment more closely to the specialty basis of service planning this second series has moved away from single interventions and diseases to include groups of interventions (terminal and palliative care), groups of diseases/problems (sexually transmitted diseases, child and adolescent mental health) and whole specialties (gynaecology, dermatology and accident and emergency services) (Table 3). Only one review, on breast cancer, is defined as a disease group. Several of the reviews however use diseases as sub-categories. Back pain is defined more by the diagnostic cluster it represents than a disease group or aetiology.

Table 3: Health care needs assessment topics

	Series 1	Series 2
Cause	Alcohol misuse Drug abuse	
Diagnosis		Low back pain
Intervention	Total hip replacement Total knee replacement Cataract surgery Hernia repair Prostatectomy for benign prostatic hyperplasia Varicose vein treatments	
Group of interventions	Family planning, abortion and fertility services	Terminal and palliative care
Disease	Renal disease Diabetes mellitus Coronary heart disease Stroke (acute cerebrovascular disease) Colorectal cancer Dementia Cancer of the lung	Breast cancer
Heretogenous group of diseases/ problems	Lower respiratory disease Mental illness	Genitourinary medicine services Child and adolescent mental health
Service/specialty	Community child health services	Gynaecology Dermatology Accident and emergency departments
Client group	People with learning disabilities	

We believe that each of the authors of the eight reviews has admirably matched the task of reviewing the components of health care needs assessment of their disease topic. Furthermore the original protocol has stood up well in its first few years. This has been so against a turbulent background in health care purchasing and a background of only slow progress in the development and availability of health care information. At the same time epidemiologically-based needs assessment has been reinforced by its overlap with other initiatives towards effective health care as well as by its uniquely wide coverage of entire diseases, groups of interventions and specialties.

References

1 Stevens A, Gabbay J. Needs assessment, needs assessment. *Health Trends* 1991; **23**: 20–3.
2 National Health Service Management Executive. *Assessing Health Care Needs*. London: Department of Health, 1991.
3 Stevens A, Raftery J. Introduction. In *Health Care Needs Assessment, the epidemiologically based needs assessment reviews. Vol. 1*. Oxford: Radcliffe Medical Press, 1994.
4 Culyer A. *Need and the National Health Service*. London: Martin Robertson, 1976.
5 *House of Commons NHS and Community Care Act*. London: HMSO, 1990.
6 *Department of Health Care Programme Approach Guidelines*. London: Department of Health, 1990.
7 Gillam S, McCartney P, Thorogood M. Health promotion in primary care. *Br Med J* 1996; **312**: 324–5.
8 Harris A. Health checks for people over 75. *Br Med J* 1992; **305**: 599–600.
9 Whitkin B, Altschuld J. *Planning and conducting needs assessments. A practical guide*. California: Sage, 1995.
10 Oregon Health Services Commission. *Prioritisation of health services*: Salem: Oregon Health Commission, 1991.
11 National Health Service Management Executive. *Local voices*. London: Department of Health, 1992.
12 Mawhinney B. Speech at the National Purchasing Conference. 13 April 1994, Birmingham.
13 Ham C. Priority setting in the NHS: reports from six districts. *Br Med J* 1993; **307**: 435–8.
14 Price D. Lessons for health care rationing from the case of child B. *Br Med J* 1996; **312**: 167–9.
15 Murray S, Graham L. Practice based health need assessment: use of four methods in a small neighbourhood. *Br Med J* 1995; **310**: 1443–8.
16 Shanks J, Kheraj S, Fish S. Better ways of assessing health needs in primary care. *Br Med J* 1995; **310**: 480–1.
17 Jarman B. Underprivileged areas: validation and distribution scores. *Br Med J* 1984; **289**: 1587–92.
18 Gunnell D, Ewing S. Infertility, prevalence, needs assessment and purchasing. *J Public Health Med* 1994; **16**: 29–35.
19 Office of Population Censuses and Surveys. *General Household Survey*. London: HMSO, 1992.
20 Martin J, Meltzer H, Elliott D. *The prevalence of disability among adults*. London: HMSO, 1988.
21 Higginson I, Victor C. Needs assessment for older people. *J R Soc Med* 1994; **87**: 471–3.
22 Advisory Group on Health Technology Assessment. *Assessing the effects of health technologies, principles, practice, proposals*. London: Department of Health, 1993.
23 Standing Group on Health Technology. *Report of the NHS Health Technology Assessment Programme 1995*. London: Department of Health, 1995.
24 Courtney P, O'Grady J, Cunnane J. The provision of secure psychiatric services in Leeds; paper I, a point prevalence study. *Health Trends* 1992, **24**: 48–50.
25 Stevens A, Gooder P, Drey N. *The prevalence and needs of people with mental illness and challenging behaviour and the appropriateness of their care*. (In press.)
26 Wing J, Thornicroft G, Brewin C. Measuring and meeting mental health needs. In *Measuring mental health needs* (eds G Thornicroft, C Brewin, J Wing). London: Royal College of Psychiatrists, 1992.
27 Sheldon TA, Raffle A, Watt I. Why the report of the Advisory Group on osteoporosis undermines evidence based purchasing. *Br Med J* 1996; **312**: 296–7.
28 Royal College of Physicians. Care of elderly people with mental illness, specialist services and medical training. London: RCP, RCPsych., 1989.
29 Bobadilla J, Cowley P, Musgrove P *et al*. Design, content and finance of an essential national package of health services. In *Global comparative assessments in the health care sector* (eds C Murray, A Lopez). Geneva: World Health Organization, 1994.

30 Brewin C. Measuring individual needs of care and services. In *Measuring mental health needs* (eds G Thornicroft, C Brewin, J Wing). London: Royal College of Psychiatrists, 1997.

31 Beech R, Gulliford M, Mays N *et al*. Renal disease. In *Health Care Needs Assessment, the epidemiologically based needs assessment reviews. Vol. 1*. Oxford: Radcliffe Medical Press, 1994.

32 Gillam S. Assessing the health care needs of populations – the general practitioners' contribution. *Brit J General Practice* 1992; **42**: 404–5.

33 Conway M, Armstrong D, Bickler G. A corporate needs assessment for the purchase of district nursing: a qualitative approach. *Public Hlth* 1995; **109**: 3337–45.

34 US Preventive Services Task Force. *Guide to clinical preventive services. An assessment of the effectiveness of 169 interventions*. Baltimore: Williams and Wilkins, 1989.

35 Williams M H, Frankel S J, Nanchahal K *et al*. Total hip replacements. In *Health Care Needs Assessment, the epidemiologically based needs assessment reviews. Vol. I*. Oxford: Radcliffe Medical Press, 1994.

36 Department of Health. *Working for patients*. London: HMSO, 1989.

37 Stevens A (ed.). Health technology evaluation research reviews. *Wessex Institute of Public Health Medicine. Vol. 2*, 1994 (248 pp) and *Vol. 3*, 1995 (285 pp).

38 Raftery J, Couper N, Stevens A. *Expenditure implications of new technologies in the NHS – an examination of 20 technologies*. Southampton: WIPHM, 1996.

39 Department of Health, Home Office. *Review of health and social services for mentally disordered offenders and others requiring similar services: final summary report*. London: HMSO, 1992. (The Reed Committee report).

40 Audit Commission. *What the doctor ordered. A study of GP fundholders in England Wales*. London: HMSO, 1996.

41 Ovretveit J. *Purchasing for health*. Buckingham: Oxford University Press, 1995.

42 Fry J. *General practice: the facts*. Oxford: Radcliffe Medical Press, 1993.

43 Chalmers I, Enkin M, Keirse M (eds). *Effective care in pregnancy and childbirth*. Oxford: Oxford University Press, 1989.

44 Neuburger H. *Cost-effectiveness register: user guide*. London: Department of Health, 1992.

45 Stevens A. *Epidemiologically based needs assessment series evaluation results*. 1993, unpublished.

46 House of Commons Health Committee. *Priority setting in the NHS: purchasing*. Minutes of evidence and appendices. London: HMSO, 1994.

47 *Purchasing Unit Review of Contracting – the third national review of contracting 1994–5*. Leeds: National Health Service Executive, 1994.

48 *Costing for contracting FDL(93)59*. Leeds: National Health Service Executive, 1993.

49 *Comparative cost data: the use of costed HRGs to inform the contracting process. EL(94)51*. Leeds: National Health Service Executive, 1994.

Child and Adolescent Mental Health

SA Wallace, JM Crown, M Berger, AD Cox

1 Summary

Introduction

This chapter reviews the need for care and services for children and young people with emotional and behavioural difficulties. Priority is given to considering those difficulties that give rise to substantial disruption of personal and social life. The emphasis throughout is on estimating need in populations, in order to make the data available in a form that will be of use to those professionals in health, social services and education who are responsible for care and service planning in child and adolescent mental health within a defined geographical area.

Health authorities are responsible for identifying the health needs of a geographically designated population and for ensuring that appropriate action is taken to meet them. Although health authorities co-ordinate child and adolescent mental health services (CAMHS), paediatric services and primary health care; other agencies provide complementary services. Social services departments are responsible for the care needs of children and adolescents and education departments provide appropriate educational facilities for all children, including those with special educational needs. Effective care in this field requires provision of services by all three major statutory agencies working in close collaboration with each other and the voluntary sector.

Child and adolescent mental health services aim to prevent, investigate, assess and treat child and adolescent mental health difficulties within the age range 0–16 years. Older adolescents who are still in full-time education may be included.

Some mental health difficulties may be dealt with effectively at the primary care level. However others, which are usually multi-factorial in aetiology and multi-faceted in their manifestations often require skilled assessment and the co-operation of different professionals and agencies for effective treatment. Child and adolescent mental health services therefore work in an interdisciplinary environment which includes professionals in the fields of psychiatry, psychology, psychotherapy, nursing, social work, education, occupational and speech and language therapy.

Epidemiological knowledge of many of the conditions has increased substantially over the past 25 years. From this it is apparent that there is a wide range of predisposing and precipitating factors which can result in an equally wide range of difficulties. Social factors are clearly implicated in the genesis and maintenance of these and in their extension into adulthood.[1] Such factors include characteristics of parents and care-givers; their mental and physical health and personalities; the quality of the parents' relationship; the style of child rearing and the contexts in which it occurs; relationships between the child and other family members; family structure and aspects of family function; life events, such as bereavements; relationships with peers; school experiences and broader environmental circumstances such as adequacy of housing.[2-7] There is also good evidence that childhood difficulties can be the precursors of adult criminality and mental disorder.[8,9]

Child and adolescent mental health is also directly and indirectly influenced by genetic factors, physical health, developmental status and educational ability. There is increasing evidence of interaction between all of these and other psychosocial factors in the genesis of mental health difficulties.[10,11]

2 Statement of the problem

Definitions

Children and young people who show patterns of behaviour, emotions or relationships that cause concern to themselves, parents, carers or teachers may be referred to CAMHS, other health services (primary care or paediatrics) or other agencies. The difficulties which precipitate such referral constitute the 'presenting problems', which may subsequently be assessed as 'clinical problems' requiring intervention. This assessment takes into account 'severity', which is a multi-dimensional concept, judged according to the criteria set out in Box 1. It may result in the diagnosis of 'disorder'. Both problems and disorders may exist in the presence of 'risk factors'.

Box 1: Dimensions used in assessing the severity of presenting problems

- Impairment: Impact on individual, carers, environment
- Age appropriateness: Departure from expected developmental course or common patterns
- Frequency
- Duration
- Persistence
- Intensity
- Extensiveness/pervasiveness
- Intrusiveness
- Manageability/controllability
- Multiple presenting problems

A **problem** is defined as a disturbance of function in one area of relationships, mood, behaviour or development of sufficient severity to require professional intervention (see Appendix II for a list of individual problems).

A **disorder** is defined either as a severe problem (commonly persistent), or the co–occurrence of a number of problems, usually in the presence of several risk factors.

Problems and disorders can include behaviour patterns and changes which are either quantitatively (e.g. tantrums or stealing) or qualitatively (e.g. autism or psychotic symptoms) different from normal, of which the latter is generally more serious. Both individual problems and disorders vary in severity.

A **risk factor** can relate to the individual child, family, environment, life events and school experience. Risk factors are such conditions, events or circumstances that are known to be associated with emotional and behavioural disorders and may increase the likelihood of such difficulties. (see Box 7 on page 16).

The association of risk factor(s) with problems or disorders implies increased severity. The prevalence of risk factors will vary from district to district (e.g. inner-city versus rural). High levels of any of the risk factors in a given population indicate the need for an increased level of provision of CAMHS.

The terms **care, service, need, demand, utilization,**[12–14] **professional** and **specialist** which are used in this chapter are defined in Appendix I.

Characterization and classification

Formal characterization and classification schemes for clinical problems and diagnoses in child and adolescent mental health have been developed for different purposes.

The proposed core data set for child and adolescent psychology and psychiatry services[15] is intended for use by professionals involved in direct patient care who are having to identify the characteristics of their patients for recording on computerized information systems. It provides a framework for detailing clinical features (problems), severity of the problems of patients and accompanying risk factors. Box 2 and Appendix II illustrate the data set.

Box 2: A clinically-based classification of child and adolescent mental health problems as derived from the Proposed Core Data Set for Child and Adolescent Psychology and Psychiatry Services

---

Problems

- Antisocial behaviour e.g. stealing, firesetting
- Problems related to school e.g. school refusal
- Problems of self-regulation e.g. tics, feeding problems
- Problems of social relationships e.g. with parents/sibs, attention seeking
- Self-harm/injury e.g. overdose
- Sexual and sex-related problems e.g. sexual offence, gender identity
- Autistic-type characteristics e.g. autism
- Psychosis-type characteristics e.g. confusion, psychotic symptoms
- Psychosomatic-related illness e.g. hypochondriasis, hysteria

Risk factors

Risk factors in the child

- Problems associated with cognition or academic abilities e.g. reading difficulty
- Personality/temperament e.g. shyness/social isolation
- Problems related to speech and language e.g. mutism, speech delay
- Physical e.g. epilepsy, head injury, chronic illness
- Sensory problems e.g. visual impairment, hearing difficulties
- Genetic condition e.g. chromosome anomaly

Risk factors in the family

- Relationship difficulty involving parent(s)/carer(s)
- Marital difficulties
- Family mental health problems
- Family physical health problems
- Abuse/neglect – physical/emotional/sexual

Risk factors in social circumstances

- Adverse social circumstances
- Life events e.g. bereavement

The tenth revision of the International Classification of Diseases (ICD 10) summarized in Box 3[16] provides a diagnostic classification which concentrates almost solely on disorders and gives indications of probable aetiology, associated factors and prognosis. For a given child or adolescent, the ICD 10 diagnosis usually encompasses several of the problems listed in the Association for Child Psychology and Psychiatric Services (ACPP) core data set (for example 'conduct disorder' might encompass aggression, defiance and truancy) though a single pattern of behaviour such as persistent firesetting may also merit a diagnosis of 'conduct disorder' (F91).

Box 3: Child and adolescent mental health disorders: international classification of diseases (ICD 10) for child and adolescent mental health

---

F90–F98   Behavioural and emotional disorders with onset usually occurring in childhood and adolescence
F90   hyperkinetic disorders
F91   conduct disorders
F92   mixed disorders of conduct and emotions
F93   emotional disorders with onset specific to childhood
F94   disorders of social functioning with onset specific to childhood and adolescence
F95   tic disorders
F98   other behavioural and emotional disorders with onset usually occurring in childhood and adolescence
F99   mental disorder, not otherwise specified

F70–F79   Mental retardation
F70   mild mental retardation
F71   moderate mental retardation
F73   severe mental retardation
F74   profound mental retardation
F78   other mental retardation
F79   unspecified mental retardation

F80–F89   Disorders of psychological development
F80   specific developmental disorders of speech and language
F81   specific developmental disorders of scholastic skills
F82   specific developmental disorder of motor function
F83   mixed specific developmental disorders
F84   pervasive developmental disorders
F88   other disorders of psychological development
F89   unspecified disorder of psychological development

In addition, some adult mental health diagnoses can become apparent in adolescents and younger children. The major groupings for these are:

F10–F19   mental and behavioural disorders due to psychoactive substance use
F20–F29   schizophrenia, schizotypal and delusional disorders
F30–F39   mood (affective) disorders
F40–F48   neurotic, stress related and somatoform disorders
F50–F59   behavioural syndromes associated with physiological disturbances and physical factors
F60–F69   disorders of adult personality behaviour

Comparing the new ICD 10 codes with equivalent ICD 9 codes or the US DSM III – R classification can be difficult but epidemiology based on any of these classifications provides useful guidance for broad categories of disorder and some specific conditions. It should be noted that the US SDM IV has been produced recently and is more comparable to ICD 10

The ICD 10 incorporates findings from recent research and is needed when planning services for populations because epidemiological data are most commonly based on such higher-order diagnoses.

3 Context

There are several clinical and organizational issues which have led to an increase in demand for child and adolescent mental health services over recent years. In young people there has been an increase in the prevalence of mental health problems such as depression, self-injurious behaviour, delinquency and substance abuse.[17] In addition legislative changes affecting social services and education have led to an increased monitoring and assessment role for these authorities. Responsibilities for treatment have increasingly passed to health services.

Other issues include the increasing recognition of the importance of certain diagnoses in this age group (e.g. pervasive developmental disorders, hyperkinetic disorders, post-traumatic stress disorders) and the need to find effective interventions for uncommon and difficult conditions (e.g. self-injurious behaviour in children with severe learning difficulties). The role of prevention has become more important, particularly the recognition of precursors of severe conditions (e.g. psychosocial adversities).[18,19] All these issues have implications for service provision and should be considered when deriving appropriate models of care to meet the specific needs for this group of children and adolescents.

The Children Act 1989

Any review of child and adolescent mental health services must consider the major service implications of the changes resulting from the Children Act (1989). Essential principles of the act emphasize the welfare of the child, responsibilities of parents and the broad obligations of local authorities to ensure that children's needs are met. The requirements of the act place new, more complex and urgent demands on CAMHS for assessment, consultation and treatment of individuals and families, as well as greater involvement in the associated administrative and legal proceedings. The service implications of the act must therefore be given full consideration in service planning for child and adolescent mental health.

Child protection

Wider appreciation of the range and nature of child abuse and neglect has led to increased pressure on local authority services to carry out monitoring and co-ordinating functions relating to child protection. The Children Act (1989) has given a new range of statutory responsibilities to local authority social services departments and this has further reduced the capacity of those departments to do therapeutic work with individual families.

The increasing demands on social service resources have led to the withdrawal of social workers from collaborative multi-disciplinary work within child mental health services. This has diminished the efficacy of collaboration between child mental health services that is essential for the welfare of children.

The 1981 Education Act

The 1981 Education Act has led to educational psychologists within school psychological services being increasingly engaged in assessments of special educational need and this has been reinforced by the 1993 Education Act.

The integration of children with mental health problems into normal school and limitations on the number of children receiving special educational needs assessments has led to more children being referred to specialist child mental health services because of emotional and behavioural problems associated with educational failure, bullying and other school-related problems. Previously, educational psychologists were more often engaged in schools and clinics in direct therapeutic programmes for individual children. More recently the Department for Education has produced guidance on the assessment of children with special educational needs and the management of children with emotional and behavioural problems in the education system.[20]

Uncommon and difficult conditions

From time to time children or adolescents require complex, long term and expensive care for uncommon conditions such as severe behaviour disorders associated with epilepsy or challenging behaviour in association with learning difficulties, or autism. There is often confusion or even conflict about the type of service required and failure to agree on the responsible authority, resulting in unacceptable delays in placing the child.

Information

Demographic and related information required to develop services and effective contracts for child and adolescent mental health will need to be obtained from a variety of different sources (Table 1). The task of collecting such data will vary between districts and depends upon quality and accessibility of both computer and library-based information.

Table 1: Source of data for child and adolescent mental health needs assessment

Local data sources	Supplementary data sources
Demographic	Ethnic composition
Ethnic composition	Hospital activity
Mortality	Morbidity
Morbidity	Social Services data
Family and socio–economic data	Socio–economic information
Police and probation	Unemployment
	Family factors
	Criminality

Data are available from a number of written and computer-based sources to provide a background picture of need for services for child and adolescent mental health. This information is by no means comprehensive and will probably require a degree of extrapolation to be used effectively.

The sources of data available can be divided into local data and supplementary data collected at a national, regional or local authority level.

Further details of these data sources can be found in Appendix III. The problems associated with collection and reliability are also identified.

Conclusion

In summary CAMHS deal with a wide range of problems and disorders from minor and self-limiting difficulties through to conditions which result in major disability and may be life-threatening. These conditions occur within a background of individual, family and social risk factors, heightened by disadvantage. There are indications that such problems and disorders are increasing. Adequate management requires a network of multi-disciplinary and flexible services.

Recent legislative and policy changes have resulted in reduced involvement in therapy and care by some professional groups which have traditionally played a major part in this service.

Against this background we proceed to develop the framework for needs assessment for child and adolescent mental health.

4 Sub-categories of child and adolescent mental health problems and disorders

Introduction

There is no single sub-categorization in use in child and adolescent mental health which has been widely adopted and which would be universally accepted by all the professional groups contributing to services. In this chapter we have divided the areas of concern into:

- clinical problems
- disorders
- risk factors.

These terms are defined on page 2.

The decision to seek help is often not taken by children or young people themselves but by parents, care givers or other adults. The type of service needed is indicated by the characteristics of the individual problems and disorders, their severity and the exact nature of the risk factors present. It should be re-emphasized that the relevant service may be required from any or all of the statutory agencies (health, social services and education).

This section describes in more detail the sub-categories of problems, disorders and risk factors. Diagnostic examples which may be of use to purchasers of CAMHS are set out with epidemiological evidence in section 5 (Boxes 5, 6 and 7 provide summaries).

Sub-categorization according to need for service

Child and adolescent mental health problems may be grouped according to whether the individual problem is likely to indicate the presence of a severe disorder. However it should be noted that severity depends not only on diagnostic classification but also on individual case characteristics (Box 1), complexity and risk factors.

Common problems with a low risk for a severe disorder

Disturbances of mood or behaviour which are quantitatively different from normal are not necessarily indicators of a severe disorder if they affect only one functional area (e.g. sleep problems or temper tantrums).

In this case they do not necessarily require management by specialist child mental health services. However if they persist or are associated with other problems such as school non-attendance, poor concentration, being bullied or teased, or multiple risk factors they may constitute a disorder and require specialist assessment or intervention.

Common disorders that are not necessarily severe

These relatively common mood and behaviour conditions usually incorporate problems that are quantitatively different from normal. They can be grouped broadly into:

- conduct disorders (e.g. problems of aggression, stealing, non-compliance)[a]
- emotional disorders (e.g. problems of anxiety, depression which do not meet adult diagnostic criteria for mood disorder)
- specific developmental disorders (e.g. problems of language and speech development). A proportion of these disorders are severe and require specialized resources, particularly those persisting beyond five years of age.

These and other disorders not infrequently co-occur in an individual and can often be dealt with satisfactorily by solo professional services. If they are persistent or there are several different risk factors present, multi-disciplinary management will be required.

Less common problems which indicate a severe disorder

Some problems are of particular importance because they point to the possibility of a severe disorder. They will usually require early, specialist CAMHS assessment. These include hallucinations, severe tics, pervasive hyperactivity, symptoms of autism and attempted suicide.

---

[a] Although some can be considered relatively mild, early onset conduct disorders and those associated with hyperactivity and poor peer relationships have a poor prognosis.

Potentially severe disorders

These comprise relatively uncommon disorders where the disturbances of mood and behaviour are qualitatively different from normal. They include:

- pervasive developmental disorders (e.g. autism)
- mental health disorders which meet diagnostic criteria for adult disorders (e.g. eating disorders, schizophrenia and mood disorders).

These disorders need multi-disciplinary specialist CAMHS assessment and may require multi-disciplinary treatment.

Risk factors

The presenting features of mental disorder in children can be associated with one or more risk factors. These add to the complexity of the condition, influence severity and so may determine the nature of the service required. Risk factors can relate to the following.

- **The child** Acute or chronic illness, specific or general learning difficulties, language and other developmental disorder.
- **The family** Parental discord, parental mental health, neglect, child abuse, criminality, economic circumstances.
- **The environment** Overcrowding, homelessness, discrimination.
- **Life events** Parental separation, acute illness, bereavement and disasters.
- **School** Bullying, victimization, inappropriate curriculum.

Multiple risk factors point to the need for specialist assessment and treatment. This is of particular importance in places where the prevalence of risk factors such as unemployment, homelessness, single parenthood and drug misuse are high. Intervention to reduce risk factors (e.g. parental postnatal depression) is an important preventive measure. In the absence of child disorder, some risk factors, such as life events, can be dealt with by the family or in primary care.

When risk factors involve relationship dysfunction, or when they are multiple (e.g. abuse and parental mental illness), multi-disciplinary assessment and intervention are likely to be needed.

Relationship between sub-categories and the Children Act 1989

The Children Act 1989 distinguishes the following.

- General needs of children for the promotion of different aspects of their development (emotional, physical, intellectual, social, behavioural and educational).
- Children 'in need' whose development would be impaired without the provision of additional resources by the local authority or health services are thought to comprise some 20% of the population.
- Significant harm which constitutes a threshold for legal action. This comprises either maltreatment by parents or caregivers, or impairment or likelihood of impairment of physical, intellectual, emotional, social or behavioural development that is attributable to the care given to the child. The child may also be beyond parental control.

The act confirms the general need for the support for all children in their development. Any child with significant or long-standing problems or with a recognized mental health disorder is 'in need'. Recent research confirms that services should address children 'in need' and not just those experiencing significant harm.[21]

Relationship between sub-categories and primary, secondary and tertiary prevention

Primary prevention aims to reduce risk factors and prevent the development of problems. This is of potential benefit to all children.

Secondary prevention aims at early detection of problems, with a view to effective intervention and prevention of recurrence or escalation. This is of benefit to children with problems and disorders, or to those exposed to risk factors which are amenable to treatment.

Tertiary prevention seeks to alleviate or minimize the disability associated with a disorder. It is of benefit to children with more serious disorders which cannot be completely eliminated.

5 Prevalence

Introduction

This section reviews the prevalence of child and adolescent mental health problems, disorders and risk factors and is set out in three main groups consistent with the definitions and sub-categories described in sections 2 and 4; clinical problems (Box 5), disorders (Box 6) and risk factors (Box 7). It is important to understand that children and adolescents presenting to services in an average district will have a variety of problems but that the majority tend to fall into two broad groups of conduct or emotional difficulties. The severity of these problems and disorders and the extent to which they are associated with risk factors will determine the level of service required for each child.

General features

Among three year olds in an urban community the prevalence of moderate to severe mental health disorders is 7% and the prevalence of mild disorders is 15%.[22] In an older population the overall prevalence of child and adolescent mental health disorders has been estimated at 12% in children aged 9–11 in rural areas (Isle of Wight) and 25% in ten year olds in inner London.[23] Amongst adolescents higher rates have been found. Although these figures seem high, in practice only about 10% of those with disorders are seen by specialist services. Referral levels are influenced by society's and primary health care professionals' perceptions of mental health problems. They are also influenced by the availability of services. As would be expected the highest proportion of referrals are for children with more severe problems.

Differences in overall prevalence between these and other surveys are usually due to the characteristics of the target sample, the sampling method, case definition and assessment procedures.[24–26]

A broad indication of overall prevalence of symptoms, disorders and risk factors is shown in Box 4.[27,28] These figures include the full range of conditions from the very mild to severe, not all of which will need specialist care.

These wide ranges of prevalence also reflect differences among populations relating to characteristics such as age, sex, ethnic distribution and whether the population is from a rural or urban setting. Other important associated factors include social class distribution and levels of deprivation. The prevalences act as a broad indication which should be adapted to meet the characteristics of particular local populations.

Box 4: Overall prevalence of child and adolescent mental health problems, disorders and risk factors

Problems	5 – 40%
Disorders	5 – 25%
Risk Factors	5 – 40%

Age and sex

In general, the prevalence of disorders is lower in the younger age group than in the older group and higher in boys than girls, although girls begin to overtake during adolescence.[29]

Ethnic differences

Data from various studies show that the prevalence and presentation of child psychiatric disorder varies between ethnic groups.[30–32] The presence and pattern of variation is not constant across subgroups or across individual disorders.

Culture can influence the presentation of psychiatric disturbance in a number of ways. Idioms of distress appear to be culturally determined in adults, such as reactive excitation in Afro-Caribbean people[33] and somatization in people of Pakistani origin.[34] Culture may also affect the presentation of emotional disorders in children and influence the way parents interpret their children's behaviour and what action they take when they consider it abnormal.

Studies in the UK suggest that children of Asian origin appear to have comparable or slightly lower rates of psychiatric disorder than white children.[31,32,35,36] There are no recent studies giving adequate estimates of prevalence across all ages in the different ethnic groups in the UK.

Incidence

Assessing incidence in child and adolescent mental health is difficult as the majority of disorders that are sufficiently severe to be dealt with by specialist services are long standing and chronic. However there are some circumstances which require an acute response (e.g. attempted suicide, drug overdose, acute psychosis and reactions to life and traumatic events, and children refusing treatment on paediatric wards). Self-harm, anorexia and child abuse carry the greatest threat to life. As numbers for suicide, death from anorexia, abuse and undetermined death are small, mortality data are not particularly helpful as indicators of need for services.

Epidemiology of problems

This is summarized in Box 5.

Nocturnal enuresis

Rutter *et al.* found 6.7% of seven year old boys and 3.3% of girls were wet more than one night a week.[37] A study of seven year old children found that 8% of children experienced night wetting.[38] A study of 14 year olds found 1.1% of boys and 0.5% of girls to be wet at least one night a week.[37]

Box 5: Prevalence of specific child and adolescent mental health problems[a]

• Nocturnal enuresis	8% of seven year old children 1% of 14 year old children
• Sleep difficulties	13% of London three year olds have persistent difficulty settling at night 14% of London three year olds wake persistently during the night
• Feeding difficulties in children	12–34% among pre-school children
• Abdominal pain without organic cause	10% in five to ten year olds
• Severe tantrums	5% of three year olds in an urban community
• Simple phobias	2.3–9.2% of children
• Tic disorders	1–13% of boys and 1–11% of girls
• Educational difficulty	specific reading retardation – 3.9% (Isle of Wight) and 9.9% (London) of ten year olds general reading backwardness – 8.3% (Isle of Wight) and 19% (London) of ten year olds

[a]Greater detail can be found in the text. Not all specific problems are represented in this box

Sleep difficulties

A study of three year old London children found that 13% had difficulty settling at night with 14% waking during the night.[22]

Feeding difficulties in young children

The prevalence of feeding problems generally among pre-school children is estimated at between 12 and 34%.[39]

Abdominal pain without organic cause

This is a common complaint in children with one study finding it occurred in 10% of 5–10 year olds.[40] Another study reported symptoms in one-third of young children persisting into adulthood.[41]

Severe tantrums in young children

Severe temper tantrums have been found in 5% of three year olds in an urban community.[22]

Simple phobias

Persistent disabling fears of specific objects or situations such as dogs or the dark occur in 2.3–9.2% of children.[26]

Tic disorders

Transient tic behaviours are commonplace among children. Community surveys indicate that 1–13% of boys and 1–11% of girls manifest frequent 'tics, twitches, mannerisms or habit spasms'.[42] Children between the ages of seven and 11 years appear to have the highest prevalence rates (5%) with the male to female ratio less than 2:1 in most community surveys (see also page 14).

Educational difficulty

In the Isle of Wight study,[43] specific reading retardation (SRR) (i.e. reading performance significantly below what could be expected on the basis of both age and intelligence) was found to affect 3.9% of ten year olds. General reading backwardness (GRB) (i.e. performance specifically below what could be expected on the basis of age) affected 8.3%. In the comparable inner London study the respective rates were double; at 9.9% SRR and 19% GRB.[44]

Epidemiology of disorders

This is summarized in Box 6.

Emotional disorders with onset specific to childhood

These disorders include anxiety and other emotional disorders not fitting adult diagnostic criteria.The estimated prevalence of emotional disorders in population-based studies varies from 4.5% of ten year old children living in small town communities (estimated from Rutter *et al.*[23]) to 5.4%[45] or 8.7%[46] for anxiety disorders, with rates of 9.9% in inner-city areas.[23] They commonly represent 25–33% of clinic attenders.

Major depression

Uncertainties surrounding the concept of depression in young people and unstandardized methods of assessment led to huge variations in the reported rates of depressive disorder. However by using standard diagnostic criteria together with more comparable methods of data collection, it has been estimated that the point prevalence for major depression is 0.5–2.5% among children and 2–8% among adolescents.[9]

Conduct disorders

The overall prevalence of conduct disorder is 6.2% among ten year olds, with the rate in boys four times higher than that in girls.[23] When similar methods were used in a relatively poor area of London the rate of conduct disorder was 10.8%.[23] 33–50% of clinic attenders have oppositional, conduct or mixed conduct and emotional disorders.

More recently the Ontario Child Health Survey has provided a comprehensive picture of conduct disorder in the general population.[47,48] The overall rate of conduct disorder in a mixed urban and rural area (5.5%) was similar to the rate reported 25 years earlier in the Isle of Wight study. Although the male to female ratio was similar, no difference between urban and rural areas was found in this part of Canada. This was interpreted as showing the importance of socio-economic status with the effect of geographical area diminishing when the degree of poverty in the different contexts was taken into account.

Box 6: Prevalence of specific child and adolescent mental health disorders[a]

• Emotional disorders with onset in childhood	4.5–9.9% of ten year olds 25–33% amongst clinic attenders
• Major depression	0.5–2.5% among children 2–8% among adolescents
• Conduct disorders	6.2–10.8% among ten year olds 33–50% amongst clinic attenders
• Multiple tic disorders	1–2%
• Obsessive compulsive disorder	1.9% of adolescents
• Hyperkinetic disorder	1.7% of primary school boys 1 in 200 in the whole population suffer severe hyperkinetic disorders Up to 17% at least some hyperkinetic problems
• Encopresis (faecal soiling)	2.3% of boys and 0.7% of girls aged 7–8 years 1.3% of boys and 0.3% of girls aged 11–12 years
• Eating disorders – anorexia nervosa	0.2–1% of 12–19 year olds 8–11 times more common in girls
– bulimia nervosa	2.5% of 13–18 year old girls and boys
• Attempted suicide	2–4% of adolescents
• Suicide	7.6 per 100 000 15–19 year olds
• Substance misuse	no figures available for effect on mental health. See text for level of use

[a]Greater detail can be found in the text. Not all disorders are represented in this box

Multiple tic disorders

Many children have simple tics (page 67) although when they are multiple and persistent, they have a serious impact on the child's education and social life. The prevalence has been estimated as 1–2% of the general population.[49]

Obsessive compulsive disorders

Figures from recent studies suggest that the weighted prevalence of obsessive compulsive disorder among adolescents is 1.9%.[50,51]

Hyperkinetic disorders

The reported prevalence of hyperactivity varies greatly. This depends predominantly on whether the problem is confined to one setting such as school or is pervasive across settings. Surveys of teachers or parents suggest figures of 17% in primary school boys.[52] The International Classification of Diseases (ICD) definition for hyperkinetic disorder includes pervasiveness and for this the prevalence is 1.7% among primary school boys. After allowing for gender differences and geographical variation, these figures imply a prevalence of one in 200 in the whole population for severe hyperkinetic disorders, with situational hyperactivity which may be part of a conduct disorder, being much more common.

Encopresis

Encopresis (faecal soiling) is found in 1.5% of children between seven and eight years of age, (boys 2.3% and girls 0.7%).[53] Rutter *et al.* found that 1.3% of boys and 0.3% of girls aged 11–12 soil at least once a month.[43]

Eating disorders

Incidence and prevalence figures for anorexia nervosa and bulimia nervosa vary among studies due to different case definitions and diagnostic criteria, as well as a lack of homogeneity among the groups surveyed.[51]

For anorexia nervosa the majority of studies reporting prevalence figures suggest that 0.2–1% of the 12–19 year old population is affected. It is 8–11 times more common in females than males.[54]

For bulimia nervosa one study suggests a reported lifetime prevalence of 2.5% among 13–18 year old boys and girls. It is more common than anorexia nervosa, peaks at about 19 years of age and is far more common in girls than boys. Bulimic patients are under-represented in clinical samples of eating-disordered adolescent patients.[55]

Attempted suicide

In US studies reported lifetime suicide attempts have been estimated at 9% of adolescents and 1% of preadolescents.[56–58] The figure for French-Canadian 12–18 year olds is 3.5%, for Dutch 14–20 year olds 2.2% and Swedish 13–18 year olds 4%. The figure for adolescents in the UK is likely to be about 2–4%.

Suicide

Suicide in childhood and early adolescence (up to the age of 15) is uncommon[59] but it increases markedly in the late teens and early twenties. In 1989 in the UK the suicide rate for children aged 5–14 years was 0.8 per 100 000 and among 15–19 year olds, 7.6 per 100 000, with suicide being more common in boys.[60]

Substance misuse

There is little information on the effect of substance misuse on the mental health of children and adolescents. Figures are generally related to the level of use of different substances. In the UK just over one-fifth of 11–15 year old children said that they had an alcoholic drink in the previous week.[61] There are high levels of regular consumption and experimentation with solvents, cannabis and more recently hallucinogens. 16% of 16 year olds regularly use solvents and illegal drugs.[62] 3–5% of 11–16 year olds have used cannabis with this figure rising to 17% in older teenagers.[63,64] However very few have been involved in regular consumption of minor tranquillizers[65–67] with less than 1% having used heroin and cocaine.[68,69]

Epidemiology of risk factors

It should be noted that overall prevalence rates for disorder reflect the impact of risk factors in individual cases. Some of the risk factors are summarized in Box 7.

Box 7: Prevalence of specific child and adolescent mental health risk factors and impact on rate of mental disorder[a]

Risk factors in child	Impact on rate of disorder
• Physical illness – chronic health problems – brain damage	three times increase in rate 4–8 times increase in rate of disorder in youngsters with cerebral palsy, epilepsy or other disorder above the brainstem
• Sensory impairments – hearing impairment four per 1000 – visual impairment 0.6 per 1000	2.5–3 times more disorder no figures but rate of disorder thought to be raised
• Learning difficulties	2–3 times increase in rate, higher in severe than moderate learning difficulties
• Language and related problems – 2%, but better methods of identifying required	four times rate of disorder

Risk factors in the family	Impact on rate of disorder
• Family breakdown – divorce affects one in four children under 16 years of age – severe marital discord	associated with a significant increase in disorders e.g. depression and anxiety
• Family size	large family size associated with increased rate of conduct disorder and delinquency in boys
• Parental mental illness – schizophrenia – maternal psychiatric disorder	eight to ten times rate of schizophrenia 1.2 to four times the rate of disorder
• Parental criminality	two to three times rate of delinquency
• Physical and emotional abuse – of those on Child Protection registers, one in four suffer physical abuse and one in eight neglect	twice rate of disorder if physically abused and thrice if neglected
• Sexual abuse – 6–62% in girls and 3–31% in boys	twice rate of disorder if sexually abused

Environmental risk factors	Impact on rate of disorder
• Socio-economic circumstances	(see text)
• Unemployment	(see text)
• Housing and homelessness	(see text)
• School environment	9% in grades one to nine are victims of bullying 7–8% of children have self-reported bullying of other children

Life events	Impact on Rate of Disorder
• Traumatic events	three to five times rate of disorder. Rises with recurrent adversities

[a]Not all specific risk factors are represented in this box

Risk factors in the child

Physical illness

- **Chronic health problems** A consistent finding in general population surveys is the increased rate of mental health and adjustment problems in children with chronic health problems, as compared with their healthy peers.[70-72] Children with chronic medical conditions and associated disability (limitations of usual childhood activities) are at more than three-fold risk for disorders and at considerable risk for social adjustment problems. Children with chronic medical conditions but no disability are at considerably less risk.[73]

  Knowledge about the causal mechanisms involved in producing the association between chronic health problems and psychological and social morbidity is incomplete. Possible mediating factors include low self-esteem, poor peer relationships and poor school performance.[73]

- **Brain dysfunction** In the Isle of Wight study the rate of disorder was increased four to eight times in youngsters with cerebral palsy, epilepsy or some other disorder above the brainstem.[74,75] Several studies indicate that brain damage or dysfunction puts children at risk for disorder in general with some increased association with hyperkinetic and pervasive developmental disorders.[74,76,77]

Sensory impairments

- **Hearing impairment** Approximately one in 1000 children has moderate to profound congenital and bilateral early onset hearing impairment,[78] rising to four in 1000 if acquired losses are included.[79] The prevalence of disorder in this group is 2.5–3 times that seen in a control group.[80-82]

- **Visual impairment** 0.3 per 1000 blind and partially sighted children at six years and 0.6 per 1000 at 11 years have been recorded in the 1958 National Child Development study. This is often compounded with additional impairments such as cerebral palsy, epilepsy and hearing impairment.[83]

Specific and general learning difficulties

The needs of children with learning difficulties have been assessed in a separate report.[84]

Children who do poorly at school, whether because of low IQ or a specific learning disorder, are at increased risk of disorder. This may be as high as 40%.[85]

The increased risk applies for a wide range of conditions, including conduct disorder,[43] delinquency,[86] hyperactivity,[87,88] depressive symptoms in adolescents,[89-95] child-reported anxiety disorders, over-anxious disorder[96] and self-reported anxiety symptoms in 11 year old girls.[97] The mechanisms by which poor school performance leads to increased rates of disorder have been investigated most fully in conduct disorder.

Language and related problems

In a longitudinal study conducted by Fundulis *et al.* the prevalence of developmental language disorder was estimated at 2%.[81] They varied in complexity and severity, the most severe requiring specialist teaching and speech therapy during school years.

However better ways of identifying children whose language impairments are truly handicapping are required. In three year olds the prevalence of behaviour problems amongst those with language delay was four times that of the general population and predicted educational difficulty at age eight.[98] Other studies have produced comparable estimates across a wide age range.[99,100]

Risk factors in the family

Family breakdown

Poor parenting, marital discord and family dysfunction have all been associated with an increased rate of disorder in children.[101] For example harsh and inconsistent parenting,[102] coercive interchanges between parent and child[103] and marital discord[104–106] are all associated with antisocial behaviour in children.

Many different factors and processes contribute to higher rates of disorder among children whose parents have separated or divorced. These include exposure to parental discord both before and after the family break up, involvement in parental disagreement and changes in family circumstances. For example if the parent with custody is emotionally distressed following the separation, then the child's behaviour may lead to critical and hostile parental responses that only serve to make the child more disturbed. These processes contribute to a prevalence of disorders as high as 80% in the first year after divorce. A US national survey showed that adolescents whose parents separated and divorced by the time the children were seven years old were three times as likely to have received psychotherapy as those from an intact family.[107]

A recent community survey of 15–20 year old girls in London confirmed that parental separation/divorce was associated with increased risk of psychiatric disorder[108] and that the quality of a mother's marriage was associated with the presence of depression and anxiety disorders.[109]

According to the General Household Survey divorce rates in England and Wales have increased markedly in the last few decades, partly as a result of legislation changes.[110] The number of persons divorcing per 1000 married people per annum rose from 9.5 in 1971, to 12 in 1980, to 13 in 1990. Haskey has estimated that if the divorce rates stabilize at the current levels, 37% of marriages will end in divorce.[111] Kiernan and Wickes suggest that divorce now affects one in four children before the age of 16.[112]

Family size

Large family size (usually four or more children) has been associated with increased rates of conduct disorder and delinquency in boys,[80,102] but not in girls.[113] The results of the Farrington and West study of inner-city boys indicate that large family size is related to antisocial behaviour and delinquency, independent of sociodemographic and parental factors.[102]

Parental mental illness

Evidence suggests that mental disorder, particularly personality disorder in either parent, is associated with increased rates of child psychopathology.[114] There is emerging evidence that specific parental psychiatric disorders are associated with increased rates of particular childhood disorders. For instance parental alcoholism and antisocial behaviour are associated with increased rates of conduct disorder and depressive symptoms and disorder (especially in the adolescent age group). Also parental anxiety disorders are associated with increased rates of anxiety disorders, particularly separation anxiety disorder (SAD).[115,116]

From a genetic perspective, children born to a schizophrenic parent have an elevated and specific risk of approximately 8–10 times for developing the disorder during their lifetime.[117]

Children whose mothers suffer from a psychiatric disorder have a 1.2–4 times increased risk of mental health problems (estimated from Rutter *et al.*[23]).

Parental criminality

Evidence suggests that parental criminality is particularly associated with disorders of conduct and delinquency in children.[101,118] The strength of the association increases if both parents have a criminal record, if they are recidivist and if their crime record extends into the period of child rearing.[119,120]

The association may be contributed to by personality abnormalities in parents such as excessive drinking or persistent aggression, modelling of deviant behaviour and child rearing that is neglectful, lacking in supervision or includes cruelty or hostility towards children.[86,119,121,122] A genetic predisposition is considered to be at least a partial explanation.[123]

Rutter has estimated that children of parents involved with crime have a 2–3 times increased risk of delinquency.[3]

Abuse/neglect

- **Physical and emotional child abuse** 4% of children up to the age of 12 are brought to the attention of professional agencies (social services departments or the National Society for the Prevention of Cruelty to Children) because of suspected abuse each year. In England in 1988, 3.5 per 1000 children below the age of 18 years were on child protection registers and more than a quarter of these were in the care of local authorities.[124] There were 24 500 additions to the register in England in 1992.[21] About one in four of those on child protection registers had suffered physical abuse and one in eight neglect. The largest proportion – one third – were subjects of grave concern, a term that often indicates another child in the family is known to have been abused. Exact figures on mortality from child abuse are unknown in the UK; a figure of at least one in 100 000 may be an underestimate.

  Young children who have been exposed to physical abuse and those exposed to neglect have twice and three times the risk of mental health problems respectively.[125]

- **Sexual abuse** The incidence of child sexual abuse is defined as the proportion of a population that has experienced it at any time during childhood. There is wide variation – from 6 to 62% in females and 3 to 31% in males – in quoted rates.[126] Categorization of sexually abusive experiences according to their severity (e.g. whether involving sexual contact) indicates that severe abuse has been experienced by 5% of women and 2% of men.[127] Children who have suffered sexual abuse have twice the risk of mental health problems.[125]

Environmental risk factors

Socio-economic circumstances

The strength of the relationship between social class and child disorder is dependent on both the measurement of social class and the measurement of disorder. If occupational prestige is used to operationalize social class, then there is a weak or non-existent relationship between it and child disorder.[22,80,128,129,130] In contrast when social class is measured in terms of economic disadvantage, then there is a strong and consistent relationship between it and child disorder.[47,48,131,132]

Unemployment

Banks and Jackson have shown that in the years after leaving school, older teenagers who had failed to find a job showed more psychiatric symptoms than those in employment.[133] The specific risk in crimes involving material gain among the unemployed suggests that the relative poverty associated with unemployment is an important mediating factor.[134]

Housing and homelessness

The links between quality of housing and child mental health has been reviewed by Quinton.[135] Living in the upper floors of high-rise accommodation, where supervision of the child's play is inevitably more difficult, is associated with depression in the mothers of young children.[136]

The deleterious effects of homelessness in families with children have been reviewed by Alperstein and Arnstein.[137] Uncontrolled studies of children living in homeless families accommodation (hotels, hostels, etc.) have revealed very high rates of developmental delay as well as emotional and behavioural problems.[138] Parents have high rates of depression.

School environment

Children spend a minimum of some 15 000 hours in school. It is therefore not surprising that experiences in school, such as bullying and pressure for academic achievement together with overall school ethos can influence the rate of childhood disorder.

Wolkind and Rutter have summarized three major aspects of schools which influence behaviour: the composition of the student body; the qualities of the school as a social organization and the efficiency of classroom management techniques.[139] If many children in the school have poor behaviour and attainment this is likely to be a consequence of poor organization and unclear discipline, lack of recognition of children as individuals, high teacher turnover and low morale.

One problem faced by children at school is bullying. A study from Norway suggests that 9% of children in grades 1–9 are victims of regular bullying and that 7–8% self-reported bullying other children.[140]

Life events

The impact of certain life events on a child or adolescent can have a varied effect on psychological well-being. Not all life events are stressors. This depends on characteristics of the event such as the social context and on the child's previous experiences.

Single traumatic events

There is evidence that life events can play a significant part in precipitating a wide range of childhood disorders.[6,7] Studies of one-off disasters which are outside normal experience indicate that they can result in reactions which are the distinctive manifestations of post-traumatic stress disorder but other disorders such as depression may also be precipitated.[2,141–143] The risk of disorder may be increased 3–5 times and rise to 100 times if there have been three recent adversities.[144]

Other life events include bereavement. In 1984 it was estimated that 3.7% of US children under the age of 18 had lost a parent.[145] Adults bereaved as children approximately double their risk of developing depression, especially if they experience a subsequent loss.[146,147] Factors that modify the outcome are reviewed by Black and include age (younger is worse), sex (girls seem more vulnerable), mode of death (sudden deaths and violent ones such as suicide or murder are associated with worse outcome) and subsequent experiences (good care lessens the risk).[148] It was concluded that bereaved children are more likely to develop disorders in childhood and in adult life, although the risk is small. Children most at risk are those bereaved young and those whose surviving parent has a prolonged grief reaction.

6 Current child and adolescent mental health services

Introduction

In this section the current variety of services available for children and adolescents with mental health problems is described. This is quantified using information from a recent national survey and highlights the different types of services available and the present staffing levels of relevant professionals.[149] There is considerable variation in available CAHMS resources in different districts.

The main service activities involve assessment, treatment, consultation/liaison, training and research. These are undertaken in community clinics, child guidance, adolescent and 'drop-in' clinics, outpatient, day-patient and inpatient services. Five types of response to child and adolescent mental health problems are described. These are:

- informal care
- primary care
- the child and adolescent mental health service: care by solo professionals
- the child and adolescent mental health service: multi-disciplinary care
- supra-district specialist multi-disciplinary care.

The pattern of care is variable across the country and several extremely successful models exist. For example solo professional care may be delivered from a unidisciplinary service or from a multi-disciplinary team. It should be noted that it is usual for any one specialist child and adolescent mental health professional to contribute to several types of care, e.g. supporting primary health care, solo, multi-disciplinary and supra-district care.

All specialist CAMHS involve professional activity outside the main professional base. This includes home and school visits for assessment or treatment purposes, attendance at child protection case conferences convened by social services and attendance at court.

It must be remembered that most child and adolescent mental health difficulties are dealt with through informal or primary care. These two areas are not covered in the recent survey and there is little additional information available from other sources.

Informal care

Single problems which are short-lived, mild and produce minimal social impairment are often dealt with entirely informally by family, friends or teachers. Examples include emotional reactions to life events, such as school entry or minor illness.

Primary care

Single problems with a low risk for severe disorder (with or without minor risk factors, see page 62) are dealt with by primary care professionals. Such problems include uncomplicated nocturnal enuresis, some general behavioural problems, feeding and sleep problems. Risk factors include overcrowding, isolation, mild parental mental health or relationship difficulties. Some general practitioners (GPs), paediatricians and health visitors have had additional specialist training in child mental health and are able to provide a service intermediate between that generally available in primary health care and specialist child mental health services.

Current status of services in primary care

Existing services vary widely across the country. Primary health care services exist in all districts, but there are often unfilled posts amongst health visitors, school nurses or community medical officers, especially in inner-city areas. Health visitors or community paediatricians with additional training in assessment and treatment of child mental health problems are present in some districts. Pilot programmes, often supported by research funds, have not always been sustained following the cessation of start-up or research funding.[150] A child development programme from Bristol is being used by many health authorities in the UK.[151] It involves a training programme for health visitors to become more aware of mental health and social problems of families they see and to help parents find their own solutions to their child rearing problems. A booklet on child mental health problems has recently been made available to all GPs in England and Wales.[152]

The child and adolescent mental health service for a population of 250 000

Solo professional care

Children with common disorders that are not necessarily severe (page 8) occurring in association with one or two risk factors need specialist care. This is often dealt with by a specialist professional (who need not be a psychiatrist) acting alone or in collaboration with primary or general paediatric care, provided that the risk factors fall within the professional's specific expertise. Examples include some children with emotional and behavioural disorders or those associated with acute and chronic physical illness, feeding difficulties and specific educational difficulty. Services may be provided by child mental health service professionals, educational psychologists and social workers or by adult psychiatrists and paediatricians who have received additional relevant training, particularly those working in the community. Solo professional care may be provided by professionals based in a multi-disciplinary group or based on a unidisciplinary service that works in a co-ordinated fashion with the multi-disciplinary service.

A less common problem which indicates a severe disorder (page 8) and common disorders that are severe and/or with multiple risk factors (page 8) will require multi-disciplinary assessment.

Multi-disciplinary care

Children with disorders comprising particularly persistent single problems, or multiple problems with several aspects of dysfunction (page 8) commonly need multi-disciplinary specialist assessment and treatment (including a child and adolescent psychiatrist), with outpatient or sometimes day unit treatment provision. Such care is also needed for children and adolescents with less common problems which indicate a severe disorder and those with potentially severe disorders (page 8). These disorders will usually be associated with major risk factors and be of long duration (three months or more). They are likely to continue if there is no intervention. For example a child with a hyperkinetic conduct disorder, who is not compliant, shows aggression to peers, has educational problems and experiences family discord, would need such management. Other examples include children and adolescents with schizophrenia or obsessive-compulsive disorders, who will require such care at some stage.

Some services run by education and social services (special schools and family units) also aim to meet this type of need. They are usually supported by specialist child mental health professionals.

Range of child and adolescent mental health services: solo professional and multi-disciplinary care

Dedicated child and adolescent mental health services within districts can include the following.

- A full range of non-residential solo professional and multi-disciplinary assessment and treatment services, including emergency cover for self-harm and other urgent conditions.
- Health day-patient facilities for children with mental health problems to complement facilities provided by educational and social services.
- A service for adolescents which may include a more directly accessible and age-appropriate component, e.g. a walk-in facility.
- Consultation and liaison services for other agencies concerned with children and adolescents. Examples include:
  a) schools, including special schools
  b) social services, especially observation and assessment centres, day nurseries and child protection services
  c) primary health care, including general practice, health visitors and school nursing
  d) specialist health services: adult psychiatry, adult clinical psychology, paediatrics including community paediatrics, child development teams and learning difficulty services
  e) voluntary agencies, e.g. NSPCC, Newpin and Home-start, and in particular, any residential or day care establishment for children and adolescents.
- Facilitation, support and training for voluntary organizations, e.g. befriending schemes and self-help groups.
- Training and collaboration with agencies listed under consultation and liaison services (a)–e) above) and to the general public.
- Administration and monitoring of the service using appropriate secretarial staff and computing.
- Admission of some children and adolescents with mental health problems to health facilities for assessment and/or treatment, e.g. paediatric wards.
- Access to services appropriate to meet the need for specialist multi-disciplinary care for populations of around one million in national centres.

Multi-disciplinary services involve closely co-ordinated assessment and treatment by fully trained child and adolescent psychiatrists, child and adolescent clinical psychologists, child psychiatric nurses, social workers and child psychotherapists, with ready access to other professional colleagues such as paediatricians, speech and language therapists, occupational therapists and teachers.

Figures for these services and the present recommended staffing levels are described on pages 24, 41 and 59.

Supra-district specialist multi-disciplinary care

Children with major mental disorders such as schizophrenia, bi-polar affective disorder, obsessive compulsive disorder, anorexia nervosa, bulimia and complex cases of autism receive care in specialist inpatient units or tertiary outpatient referral centres, with moderate to close geographical accessibility.

Severe conduct disorders also receive this provision if there is an associated mood disorder or self-injurious behaviour or factors such as epilepsy, requiring inpatient assessment. However children with uncomplicated severe conduct disorders requiring residential provision may be placed in a residential school or social service units with education.

National centres

Highly specialized services based around multi-disciplinary assessment and treatment are used for a small number of children with complex neuropsychiatric problems associated with severe behavioural disturbance, those with severe behavioural disorders who require containment within secure units and those with certain rare conditions such as gender identity problems or profound sensory problems with associated psychiatric disorders.

Current service status for child and adolescent mental health services

The following information is a summary of the findings from a recent survey of services for the mental health of children and young people in the UK.[149] It looks at purchasing authorities and the various aspects of child and adolescent services, including community-based care, inpatient and special units, day treatment services, clinical psychology services, paediatric services, social services, education and the non-voluntary sector. Further details including figures from the survey are described in Appendix IV.

- The matching of provision to local needs has hardly begun and purchasers are still dependent on what the local units say they are providing.
- The specialist child and adolescent mental health services are largely delivered from a community base, by means of inter-disciplinary teams. Psychiatrists and psychiatric social workers are almost universally members of these teams, although the number of social workers has reduced in the past three years. In this period there has been both expansion and reduction of services in different parts of the country. However the overall provision of service has remained roughly the same. Changes appear to have been somewhat arbitrary, often based on local enthusiasm or on enforced reorganization in local authority services. Numbers of staff and the range of skills available vary widely. There is little input from the education sector.
- There is major variation in the distribution of child and adolescent psychiatrists across the country and in the type of work they undertake.
- Clinical psychology is a growing profession, working increasingly from an independent base. Clinical psychologists still work mainly with the child and adolescent mental health teams, but they also provide direct solo and consultative services to acute and community services in other parts of the NHS, to social services and other agencies.
- Almost two-thirds of mental health services for children now employ a psychiatric community nurse. However few nurses have training in children's and adolescents' psychiatric care and many seem to rely on skills acquired on short random courses.
- Many inpatient units, including former regional adolescent units, are experiencing problems particularly with respect to the new system of contracting for services.
- More children with emotional and behavioural disorder present to paediatricians than to any other profession. Paediatricians' training in the main does not prepare them for this and they would welcome further opportunities to gain relevant experience.
- Local education authorities are greatly concerned with emotional and behavioural difficulties in their pupils.
- Behaviour support services, as currently provided in three-quarters of local education authorities, include assessment of the educational needs of pupils with severe behaviour problems, but infrequently no relevant medical contribution is included. Special schools for children with emotional and behavioural difficulties report that few pupils have statements in which therapeutic help is specified, although the head teachers consider that nearly half of all pupils would benefit from such help.

- The educational psychology services state that part of their function is to work with individual children whose behaviour is causing concern, but most find that assessment activity takes up most of their time. Although all services agree that joint work should make a major contribution to the management of problems in children, education authorities limit their staff resources for collaborative work.
- Social services departments concentrate resources on children in need, many of whom have serious emotional and behavioural problems. They report unsatisfactory access to specialist expertise in children's mental health from the NHS.
- The voluntary sector plays a large part at primary care level, particularly in providing services such as counselling. They often take self-referrals. Voluntary organizations also act as a filter to specialist mental health and social services. Since the NHS mental health services accept self-referrals less and less, the voluntary services may be filling a gap in provision. Some voluntary services such as the NSPCC, Barnardos and NCH offer particular expertise of value also for secondary and tertiary provision.

Assessment, management and treatment procedures

To respond to the mental health needs of their patients, child and adult mental health services initiate a variety of assessment, management and treatment procedures. The diversity of these activities is illustrated in Box 8 which shows the broad categories of treatment, investigations and case management undertaken by services. Because of the complexity of needs dealt with, several of these investigative, treatment and care-related procedures will be implemented concurrently or sequentially during an individual care episode.

Box 8: Range of assessment, management and treatment procedures

Assessment
Limited involvement
Individual treatments – child/young person
Physical illness management
Group procedures – child/young person
Work with parents
Family/marital therapy
Community visits
Collaborative work (non-team/service member)
Referral out of team/unit for opinion/non-collaborative management during episode
Tests and investigations
Reports
Attending meetings and formal procedures
Consultation
Status change/extension during episode (e.g. switch to inpatient care)
Clinical trial/experimental interventions

Source: [15]

The information in Box 8 does not detail many of the more specific forms of treatment, investigations and other procedures that have been developed, for instance the variety of medications to deal with anxiety or hyperactivity or the variants of family, psychotherapeutic and behaviourally-based therapies among others. Further it does not list the activities aimed at larger scale prevention or those aimed at the enhancement of practice and the quality of services through training of both service staff and the staffs of other agencies.

Finally services are also involved in the conduct of clinical and service-relevant research recognized as important activities for child and adolescent mental health services.

The activities listed in Box 8 can be grouped into a number of major forms of service which are undertaken in fully resourced and staffed services.

Assessment

Child and adolescent mental health services provide a number of specialist assessments as a basis for treatment or for other purposes:

- The establishment of 'caseness'. The referrer wishes to establish whether the individual has problems that constitute a mental health disorder, but does not request the assessor to undertake treatment.
- Second opinion requests. The referrer requests confirmation of a diagnosis and will deal with the ensuing needs.
- Conventional assessments to inform treatment and management within the service. Such assessments can be fairly rapid or may need to develop over time. Sometimes these include the clinical assessment of complex problems such as neuropsychiatric disorders.
- Complex assessments are those usually carried out for the courts, social services or other agencies. They require detailed information, usually culminating in a long report and consume substantial amounts of professional time. These assessments may not lead to treatment by the service. Most commonly requests for such assessments are from social services or the courts and arise because of proceedings under the Children Act. (Adequate assessment involves not just formal diagnostic categorization of the disorder, but full formulation of the problems including establishment of predisposing, precipitating and maintaining factors, prognosis and plans for intervention.)

Consultation/liaison

Parents, carers and agencies involved in looking after children and young people often need to discuss issues related to referral, diagnosis and management with specialist mental health services without wishing the case to be taken on by the child and adolescent mental health service. The processes of consultation are well-established.[153] In these instances the 'consultant' works with staff who have direct contact with the patient or patients. The individual patient may not be seen during the consultation, although he or she may be known to the service. Such work can be a more effective use of resources in dealing with the individual child or groups of children. In these instances the consultant works with staff (e.g. in schools or children's homes) who have direct contact.

Some services also provide psychiatric, psychological and psychotherapeutic input to paediatric and other wards to assist in diagnosis, management or treatment.[154]

Treatment and management

It is not always easy to differentiate assessment and treatment since the act of referral or even the recognition that a referral to specialist services is needed can initiate changes, as can the first meetings with clinic services even when no systematic attempt is made to produce change.

Interventions involve the use of recognized procedures aimed at removing, reducing or containing symptomatology and achieving a more constructive adaptation and healthy development. Since the symptomatology is invariably expressed in or influenced by the family or school, work with other family members and teachers is essential. Other adults and children may also be involved e.g. club leaders and class peers. There are several further goals of intervention as follows.

- To help clients and relevant responsible adults develop an understanding of the problems and the mechanisms of treatment so that they can anticipate and avert relapse.
- To deal with the symptomatology and contributing context in such a way that interference with the ordinary life and on-going functioning of patient, family or other carers is minimized.
- To prevent the emergence of other difficulties.
- To enhance the quality of psychosocial functioning, present and future.

Emergency services

Many child and adolescent psychiatrists and some multi-disciplinary teams provide emergency input to hospital A and E and paediatric departments dealing with psychiatric emergencies in children and young people. Most commonly these are instances of self-harm or attempted self-harm.

Training

Part of the skill and knowledge base of mental health professionals can be taught to individuals (for instance teachers, nursery staff and social workers) who have non-specialist responsibilities for dealing with mental health needs. Requests for training will sometimes emerge following consultation or may arise directly from other agencies such as day nurseries, social services or schools. Training has both a reactive and a proactive intent: to deal with current difficulties and to make those being trained better able to prevent the emergence or recurrence of problems and disorders.

Professional education and continuing professional development

In common with other professional groups, child and adolescent mental health professionals are responsible for training entrants to their and other disciplines through both formal academic teaching and supervised clinical practice. Training schemes are commonly linked with university academic departments.

Professionals with academic posts usually carry responsibility for training in conjunction with honorary NHS sessional contracts.

Research

Many services undertake research into treatment and other aspects of service delivery, both to enhance practice and improve organizational processes. Job descriptions commonly include provision for research.

Academic psychiatry and psychology departments also play a central role in supporting research carried out by NHS staff as well as initiating and undertaking clinical and academic research of direct relevance to NHS CAMHS.

7 Treatment effectiveness of mental health services for children and young people

Treatment and outcomes: an overview

Mental health services for children and young people provide a variety of assessments, treatments and other interventions for individuals, families and groups, as well as teaching, training and research. It is difficult to demonstrate conclusively a cause and effect relationship between interventions and changes, particularly with children and families with severe or long-standing difficulties.

In the introduction to a recent collection of papers on the topic of 'Psychosocial treatment research' in child and adolescent mental health, Hibbs states that:

... except in the instance of attention deficit hyperactivity disorder (ADHD), there is little research to corroborate the efficacy of well-defined treatments ... behavioural, cognitive-behavioural, and combined pharmacological/psychosocial/parent training... And there is even greater dearth of research for treatments such as psychodynamic, interpersonal, group, family therapy, and eclectic approaches, which are commonly used in clinical settings and by private practitioners. (page 2)[155]

The evaluation of treatments for children and young people with mental health needs is probably more complex than evaluations in other conditions. Some of the reasons for this are discussed later.

Evidence is accumulating for the efficacy of a range of treatments and clinicians working in mental health services for children, young people and their families will identify many clients who they feel have benefited enormously from the therapeutic interventions provided by the service. Likewise there will be teachers, social workers, health visitors and other professionals who will attest to the ways in which the advice and support provided by these services have been of benefit to them and their clients. There will also be others whose response will be less positive and yet others where the impact of the service has been negligible or who will report that intervention made things worse. In this respect child and adolescent mental health services are similar to many other clinical services.

The absence of a substantial body of information or strong evidence of the effectiveness of psychological and pharmacological treatments for children and young people is well recognized and of general concern. This has been of such importance as to have led, at the request of the Federal Government in the US, to the establishment of a task group by the National Institute of Mental Health with the brief to expand research on 'psychosocial treatments' of young people.[155] A need for similar action exists in this country.

Consequently what is possible at the present time is a limited evaluation of the effectiveness of the treatments that services offer although, even here it will be seen that while the conclusions provide good grounds for optimism, there is much that still has to be done to establish that treatments meet strong criteria for effectiveness.

This section focuses on treatment outcomes rather than the effectiveness of services. It examines some of the major reasons for the present uncertainty and provides an update of the evidence regarding the treatment of the major psychological and psychiatric disorders and an overview of the current state of treatment research.

Evaluating interventions

Research on the effectiveness of interventions for mental health needs in children and young people is complex. In order to undertake controlled studies with random assignment of cases – the standard methodology – potentially influential variables such as the severity of the condition, economic status of the family, ability, ethnicity, marital status of carers, mental ability of the child, age and sex, all need to be taken into account. Few researchers have the resources to assemble the very large samples of patients needed to achieve such control, so that research on treatment tends to involve small groups with resulting limitations on the generalizability of the findings.

Psychological treatments are also very difficult to standardize: the therapist follows a general approach but has to tailor this to the idiosyncrasies of the individual patient and family. In some cases treatment may be given by the parent on the instruction of the clinician so that procedural uniformity may be difficult to achieve. Added to this is the tendency for placebo and placebo-like effects to be very influential in research involving psychological or psychopharmacological treatments.[156] Given such complexity and the variety of human individual differences, it is also difficult to mount replication studies to check on initial findings.

These sorts of difficulties are not unique to mental health investigations but are particularly salient and intrusive in research involving multi-faceted social and psychological processes, especially with children and young people.

Consequently evidence for the efficacy of interventions is accumulated through a series of studies, each having some limitations, but each nevertheless contributing to an understanding of treatment effectiveness. Authoritative, independently assessed review articles which contain detailed methodological critiques of a large number of studies bring this together. Examples include the effects of child psychotherapy, as reported in 43 separate studies, and documented by Barnett, Docherty and Frommelt.[157] Pfeiffer and Strzelecki have reviewed the outcomes reported in 34 studies of residential and inpatient psychiatric treatment.[158] Graziano and Diament reviewed 155 empirical studies of the effects of training parents of children presenting with behaviour problems in behaviour management techniques.[159] Allen *et al.* examined 904 child behaviour therapy studies for evidence that the authors had attempted to check that effects generalized beyond the treatment programme.[160]

It is from reviews such as these that the emergent views of the effectiveness of different treatment procedures or treatments for particular conditions arise: that is, from publications that have taken due account of the methodological constraints of the contributing studies.[a]

Reviews of studies of clinical effectiveness then serve to inform and guide practice. They cannot however either determine what is done or even ensure favourable outcome in the individual case.

Treatment trials and service effectiveness

Controlled trials with random allocation of cases to different treatments require selection of cases, standard procedures and intensive monitoring of impact. Because of these and other special characteristics of the research it is difficult to extrapolate conclusions from such trials to likely outcomes in clinic populations or for clinic services: patients cannot be selected and the therapists are applying a wider range of treatment procedures to a symptomatically and otherwise heterogeneous client group.

Furthermore in clinical trials patients or their carers may be volunteers or agree to participation in research trials. In child and adolescent mental health services the identified patient and family may not have actively sought or even be willing participants in treatment. Children and young people are brought to the service, sometimes reluctantly, by family members or other carers. The family itself may have had to be persuaded or even, on occasion, coerced to attend because of a threat of expulsion from school or the concerns of social services or other agencies.

For these and other reasons, as Weisz and Weiss have suggested, it is difficult to generalize from research treatments to clinic service treatments.[161]

In a more recent analysis of the limited success of clinic services as contrasted with the outcomes of research treatments carried out in academic centres, Weisz *et al.* found only three of ten possible reasons were supported by their analysis of the research literature.[162] First research therapy that is structured is more successful than the unstructured approaches that tend to be used in clinics. Second the research treatments that are more successful tend to be focused and specific. As such treatments tend to be easier to implement

---

[a] In the main, the information on the effectiveness of mental health interventions in children and young people presented in later sections of this chapter is based on the conclusions drawn from such reviews. In those instances where this is not the case, conclusions are based on the views of clinicians who are themselves commonly involved in treatment research and who would in any event be taking account of the reviews and related literature.

and control for research purposes and may account for the better outcomes of controlled laboratory studies. Third behavioural treatments tend to have greater effect sizes than non-behavioural interventions.

These authors go on to note that if 'effect sizes are generally higher for behavioural methods... and if behavioural methods are more common in research therapy... then the superior effects of research therapy might be attributable to differences in methods of intervention.' (page 96)

Weisz *et al.* in trying to account for differences in effect sizes and noting the limitations of their approach, nevertheless found that the epoch of the study, severity of condition, the clinical setting, therapist experience, training and caseload and the length of therapy did not emerge as significant influences.[162]

Constraints on outcome

Apart from the efficacy of treatments the factors that influence outcome in the individual case are many, some facilitating and others constraining the effectiveness of services. Not all of these are under direct control of the service.

Procedures for management and treatment are in many cases not carried out by health professionals but others, particularly parents and teachers. The impact of interventions is therefore dependent on, among other factors, parent/carer compliance with the regimen. This can involve bringing the child to clinic appointments, sometimes on a weekly basis for therapy sessions; rigorous data collection (for instance on tantrum frequency); carrying out of precise procedures of monitoring and intervention at home. It may require the involvement of the whole family, sometimes over an extended period. The patient may also have several sibs so that the 'parent as therapist' is implementing the treatment in a family context of competing demands.

Apart from the critical role of parents as facilitators of the intervention processes for their children, parents have their own needs. These may require the attention of services and should also be taken into account in the evaluation of treatment outcomes as the unmet needs of parents may prevent effective interventions with their children.[163]

Participants in treatment (children and parents) may have firm ideas about the appropriateness of the treatment proposed which can limit compliance. Treatments that include medication may be resisted, even though there is increasing evidence of efficacy in specific conditions. Carers may have particular expectations, for instance that the child will be offered dynamic psychotherapy and so resist other treatment.

Many external factors confound treatment effectiveness. Concurrent factors such as inadequate housing can indirectly maintain and prolong the child's problems. In this case improvement may depend on external agencies over which health services have little if any control. Similar circumstances arise in the treatment of school phobia where the school for organizational or other reasons may not be able to participate actively in the treatment programme.

It is against this background that we proceed to examine the empirical evidence for treatment effectiveness.

Research and clinical findings

Reviews of treatment research can be major condition-centred (i.e. following ICD categories), problem-centred (e.g. the treatment of aggression), procedure-centred (e.g. analytical psychotherapy), event-centred (e.g. post-traumatic reactions) or quality of life centred (e.g. focusing on impact on family and others as well as the index individual).

As noted earlier there is as yet no evidence of high probability outcomes for the interventions provided by CAMHS. Instead there are individual case reports and a number of controlled studies in the literature on the effectiveness of psychosocial interventions, the conclusions of which support the use of some of the procedures. The ways in which they are used will be discussed at the end of this section.

While there are many case reports recording the success of specific interventions with children and young people, some of which incorporate methodologies such as single case designs, it is recognized that such studies are limited in terms of the generalizations they permit. For instance a recent report on the effectiveness of cognitive-behavioural interventions with and without pharmacotherapy, in cases of obsessional compulsive disorder supports the effectiveness of this approach but is based mainly on treatment reports of single cases.[164] Single-case studies and clinical reports will not be considered further here, even though they frequently provide an inspiration for clinicians, especially when treatment options are otherwise limited.

This section is based on reviews of empirical research on psychological and pharmacological treatments of child and adolescent mental health disorders, as these are the basis of much epidemiological research. It is intended to provide a broad perspective on psychosocial treatments rather than a detailed review of all studies or all types of intervention for specific conditions.

General evidence

Overviews of the controlled studies are at present analysed in terms of the effect sizes from meta-analyses. Taken overall the outcomes of psychological treatments (collectively called the psychotherapies, encompassing behavioural and psychodynamic, as well as other approaches) of children and adolescents 'indicate that psychotherapy is better than no treatment, that the magnitude of improvement in juveniles parallels the treatment gains reported in adults, and that differences between treatment tend to favour behaviour therapy', the latter including cognitive treatments.[163] These outcomes have however to be qualified. First according to Kovacs and Lohr, many of the studies did not include clinically referred children. Second they note that the positive outcomes for behavioural treatments may reflect a form of criterion contamination in that the treatment targets were similar to the outcome measures – when this effect is eliminated, the superiority of behavioural treatments no longer holds.

The meta-analysis studies also mask significant differences in outcomes between younger children (4–12 year olds) and teenagers (13–18 year olds).[163]

Conduct/antisocial disorders

Earls notes that chronic conduct disorders carry a high social cost and are among the most resistant to intervention.[165] Treatment needs to be focused on the individual, family or wider group depending on the outcome of assessment. Individual-only treatment is unlikely to have an impact.

Recent research is beginning to identify successful approaches to treatment.

According to Earls community-based approaches and those that involve social problem solving skills training have been shown to have beneficial effects.[165] Medication has yet to be demonstrated to have any specific value, apart from its use where other conditions coexist with the conduct disorder.

However in aggressive children who are hospitalized, treatment with lithium appears to have some beneficial effects according to the findings of a recent double-blind trial.[166] Alessi et al. suggest that there is increasing evidence for the usefulness of lithium in a number of childhood and adolescent disorders.[167]

Kazdin et al. have demonstrated the usefulness of parent training and problem solving skills training in the treatment of severe antisocial behaviour.[168]

Predictors of treatment drop-out have been described.[169] These include having a very severe form of the disorder, a mother undergoing severe stress and high levels of socio-economic disadvantage. This information enables procedures to be developed which reduce drop-out and so increase the chance of improved outcomes.

In their review Offord and Bennett also conclude that there is as yet little effective treatment for these disorders.[170] This is of major concern because of the associations with difficulties in later life.

Affective disorders

The treatment of affective disorders in children and young people tends to follow the pattern of treatment of such disorders in adults, but with greater emphasis on the involvement of the family and less frequent use of medication.

The outcome of treatment for depression has been recently reviewed.[171-174] Reynolds has also reviewed studies of depression in adolescents.[175] There is some, albeit weak, evidence that psychological approaches can have a beneficial effect on mild forms of depression, though the main thrust in treatment research has been in the use of anti-depressant medication. To date there is little firm evidence that such medication works better than placebo in children or adolescents with major depression.[171,175] As depression in children is a recently recognized condition, it is suggested that it is still too early to make firm judgements regarding all forms of treatment.[174]

Anxiety disorders

There have been a number of recent reviews and overviews of the treatment of anxiety disorders in children and young people.[176-180] One reviewer[176] recommends the use of pharmacological treatments for these disorders, while others are consistent in the conclusion that as yet, no approach to treatment is well substantiated, other than that for obsessional compulsive disorder (see below). Bernstein and Borchardt discuss treatments for anxiety.[177] They note a number of studies using different forms of medication and suggest the use of, as well as further research into the effectiveness of different medications. Klein believes that behavioural treatments are rational since rapid improvements are noted clinically in many children when such treatments are instituted.[180]

Post-traumatic stress disorder and attempted suicide

There is no research involving controlled trials but there are well documented and commonly applied management procedures. In the case of attempted suicide, for example, there needs to be a rapid response from the service in order to engage the young person and family and initiate treatment.

Anorexia nervosa and bulimia nervosa

Anorexia is a life threatening condition.[181] A variety of treatment approaches is available and should include family and individual psychotherapy, behavioural treatments, availability of inpatient treatment or occasionally medication.

Bulimia is a more recently studied condition.[181] Although there has been a substantial amount of treatment research the reported studies are methodologically inadequate so there is as yet no firm evidence of specific benefits.

Obsessive compulsive disorders

The treatment of obsessive-compulsive disorders in children closely follows that in adults. Although the efficacy of behavioural approaches is well documented in adult patients it has yet to be demonstrated through controlled studies with children.[182] Medication with clomipramine is effective, though it is likely to be needed for a prolonged period.[182,183] There are no systematic comparisons of drug versus behavioural approaches. As noted earlier the use of cognitive-behavioural treatments alone or in combination with medication in the treatment of obsessional compulsive disorder is supported by some.[164]

Attention deficit and overactivity

These syndromes are characterized by frequent co-morbidity and psychosocial adversity.[184] The most effective symptomatic treatment is stimulant medication,[184,185] though the benefits are lost on cessation of treatment.[186] Therefore medication should be accompanied by treatment of other difficulties, such as school learning, social relationships and self-esteem. DuPaul and Barkley reviewed the combined use of behavioural and pharmacological therapies and noted the added benefits for some children treated this way.[187]

Tic disorders

Psychosocial interventions involving education about the disorder as well as support, form the core of treatment, with pharmacological treatment being used in the more severe cases. While there is consistent evidence of response to medication in the majority of those treated, side-effects can be intrusive. Cognitive, behavioural and other psychotherapeutic treatments show some evidence of effectiveness, but the findings need to be replicated in further studies.[188]

Feeding and sleeping disorders in young children

There are well documented procedures for treating feeding difficulties in young children, but as Skuse notes, the main evidence on effectiveness derives from successfully treated single cases.[189]

Difficulties of getting to sleep and night waking are the most common forms and tend to be responsive to simple behavioural management.[189] There are well-tried treatments for other conditions that arise during sleep but as yet without documented controlled trials of their effectiveness.

Disorders of attachment

These problems, usually in the relationship between mother and infant or child, have been treated in various ways commonly involving the mother–child pair in the programme. There is however no systematic treatment research that provides a clear basis for specific interventions.[190]

Autism, learning difficulties and related developmental disorders

Although the core problems in these conditions are not modifiable to a major extent, they may require long-term intervention from mental health services. Of particular importance are programmes that deal with secondary behavioural or emotional disorders and training in social skills. The needs of individuals with autism and their families have been well documented and the overall management programme involves provision for medical care, appropriate education, family support and where necessary, focused treatment with speech and language, social skills or other therapies. Pharmacological treatments are as yet without major value but are seen as potentially helpful adjuncts to the overall treatment programme.[191]

Bed wetting and faecal soiling

Nocturnal enuresis has inspired a wide variety of treatments including surgery, medications, night waking and the use of a special alarm which is the only procedure known to cure the condition.[60] Cure rates average about 80% using the alarm, but it can be a difficult procedure to maintain. While relapses do occur, they do so with lesser frequency than when cessation of wetting is accomplished by other means. Medication has short-term benefits in nocturnal enuresis. Encopresis requires both medical and psychological management.

Schizophrenia

Schizophrenia is an appropriate diagnosis for a few older children and adolescents. As with the adult form, it is an incurable or recurrent condition, but persistent symptoms can be controlled with appropriate treatment. The major concerns relate to the consequences of the disorder for the child and family. As there is little evidence on the treatment and outcome in children and young people, Werry and Taylor propose that the efficacy of treatment is assumed to be much the same as for adults.[192] Pharmacotherapy is a major component of treatment and there is substantial evidence that it is 'very helpful in schizophrenia in adults'.[192] Work with the child's family may be important for prevention of relapse.

Some psychologically based approaches to management and treatment in adults appear to have value but their efficacy with this group still requires much stronger support from adequate research. Consequently there is little basis for generalizing to younger age groups.

Atypical psychosexual development

There are several treatment approaches for children and young people with atypical sexual development that report some successful results but there are no trials of treatment sufficient to enable firm conclusions to be drawn.[193]

Somatic diseases and disorders combined with chronic physical illness

The risk of psychological and psychiatric disorders is doubled in populations with major chronic illnesses.[194] The nature of the disorders is much the same as in individuals without the illness so treatment approaches follow those adopted for patients without physical illness. There are no controlled trials of treatment procedures for combined psychological and physical disorders. Specific approaches are available for pain management and to help children cope with medical procedures.

Physical and sexual abuse

The treatment of individuals who have been abused is complex and needs to take account of a multiplicity of factors. The aims are to deal with any current disorder resulting from the abuse and to prevent future mental ill-health. Removal of the child to a hospital, residential unit or other place of safety may be required. The treatment approach depends on the extent to which the factors that led to the abuse can be identified and the willingness of the individuals concerned to participate in treatment. Work with parents and families is essential if children are to remain at home. There are indications that successful behaviour modification, such as anger management in the abusers, can be beneficial for some children.[195] Individual dynamic psychotherapeutic approaches are also used.

O'Donohue and Elliott have reviewed reports of studies using psychotherapeutic procedures with sexually abused children.[196] Systematic studies have begun to delineate some of the characteristics of families which are not treatable, so that service resources can begin to be focused more efficiently.[197]

Smith and Bentovim note that an increasing number of treatments for sexual abuse are being investigated but there are insufficient controlled studies so that conclusions about the effectiveness of treatments are still premature.[198]

Prevention

Prevention of child and adolescent mental health difficulties is important because of the risk of problems continuing into adult life. Recent reviews of prevention are provided by Cox[18] and Graham.[19]

While much research has focused on treatment or other aspects of disorders, comparatively little attention has been given to prevention. There is, however, an increasing interest in prevention, particularly on a more 'macro', community level. Conceptual and methodological frameworks for the evaluation of preventive interventions have been elaborated.[199] Systematic studies in the US are also beginning to show that preventive interventions can have a beneficial impact on different aspects of the behaviour and mental health of children and young people. Interventions include helping them to resist drug taking and to deal with such stressful transitions as school transfer.[199] Recent reviews of research on the prevention of physical abuse and neglect[200] and sexual abuse[201] have also shown that some benefits can be achieved through focused prevention programmes. One major study in the UK provided encouraging results for a school-based psychotherapeutic intervention for children with behaviour problems.[202]

Preventive interventions are clearly possible and of great potential benefit, and given the assumption that such interventions can lead to the reduction in the prevalence and incidence of disorders, evaluative studies appear to be well worth supporting, particularly in communities or contexts where the risks for emotional and behavioural problems are known and high.

Criteria for judging treatment research in child and adolescent mental health services

Methodological difficulties are common in all clinical research.[203] Since the earlier reviews of treatment for children with emotional and behavioural disorders,[204] some of the major advances that have taken place involve methodological refinements and the consequent introduction of new criteria to be used in the evaluation of studies and outcomes.

Criteria for judging the efficacy of treatment have become increasingly sophisticated and complex. Although some of these criteria are condition specific – for instance in autism the underlying problem is not curable but change in major secondary symptoms is a realistic goal – there are general criteria that are now seen as core requirements.

Among the changes and improvements noted by Kovacs and Lohr has been the introduction of treatment manuals which are aimed at clearer specification of how the treatment should be implemented. Criteria to assess improvement 'have become more specific and multidimensional' and definitions solely in terms of clinicians' global judgements replaced by more objective measures involving direct observations and 'operationally defined scales' (pages 14–15).[163]

It is also recognized that it is now no longer sufficient to report statistical significance. Treatment research must also demonstrate that the changes have clinical significance, and that there is an impact on daily life, adaptation and relationships. There is also the need to demonstrate that treated clients move much closer to, or into the 'normal' range on assessment instruments. Other criteria include:

- a range of different methods for appraising outcome, rather than a single procedure (this includes evaluating process or relationships and not just symptomatology)
- a number of judges of outcome, each with a differing perspective
- assessments of functioning, both pre- and post-intervention which monitor 'internal changes' (both physiological – if appropriate – self-perceptions, and behaviours)
- statistical or other controls for co-morbidity

- assessments of stability of changes over time, since benefits are often not apparent for some time after the intervention
- monitoring of generalizability of improvements across situations (e.g. home and school)
- evidence that the intervention is better than no treatment
- evidence that the intervention is more cost-effective than other procedures
- evidence that there are minimal harmful side-effects.

Treatment research and service implications

The clinical and research literature on treatment, consisting of case reports, small-scale studies and controlled trials, constitutes the major resource for innovation and the modification of service interventions and practice. It is however not realistic to assume that favourable outcomes reported in the literature will invariably translate into positive outcomes in practice.

The nature of individual differences in the aetiology, presentation and external circumstances of children and young people, as well as the resources of services, militate against a simple formula for linking need, intervention and outcome in clinical practice. Even impressive interventions such as the use of medication in children with attention deficit and hyperactivity do not succeed in every case: an appreciable number of children are not helped by the treatment. Indeed, prediction of outcome in the individual case, given the complexity of aetiology, presentation and individual circumstance, is hazardous and a challenge for future research.

Furthermore it is necessary for findings to be replicated in independent studies. Much research emanates from the US and differences in the regulation of medication, the contexts of clinical practice, and the clinical populations studied make it hazardous to extrapolate the results to the UK population.

There can also be a major time lag between the identification of a psychological treatment procedure that shows promise and its systematic introduction in services. This is partly because suitable cases appear intermittently in services and the procedures, for instance cognitive-behavioural treatment, can require specialized training and a period of ongoing supervision.

Conclusion

At present there are few examples of child and adolescent mental health treatment that can unequivocally demonstrate their effectiveness. However substantial progress has been made in identifying the range of interventions that have the potential to benefit children and young people with mental health problems and disorders and their families. This range of treatments should be potentially available to all children and adolescents.

Klein has asserted that '...clinicians cannot await the scientific verdict to care for children who seek treatment.' (page 367).[180] The research underlines the importance of careful monitoring of progress in individual cases undergoing treatment. There should be a preparedness to change the approach where the current procedures are ineffective. The critical importance of controlled treatment trials lies in the inspiration, opportunities and direction they give to clinicians in selecting procedures likely to be the most efficacious. The effectiveness of services is then dependent on their having the resources and the skill to exploit the treatment research literature.

8 Models of care

Principles

There are several important principles which need to be accepted in developing models of care in child and adolescent mental health.

The majority of child and adolescent mental health problems can be dealt with in primary care

Many mental health problems in children and young people can be dealt with at the primary care level. As with other disciplines this can only be achieved if the health professionals at this level have adequate training in the subject and maintain their skills through continuing education. This will usually be provided by specialist child mental health professionals. Primary care teams may identify members who will develop particular expertise in this field, though all team members must be able to recognize mental health problems in children at an early stage.

The primary care team should have ready access to colleagues with additional training such as school nurses or community paediatricians, who may be team members.

The primary care team can only function satisfactorily if it is confident that specialist help is readily available when needed through local CAMHS. Primary care staff should recognize the limits of their competence and not retain responsibility for the care of children whose problems are beyond their experience.

Specialists should provide support to other groups

Specialist child and adolescent mental health professionals should support and promote the activities of primary health care, other professionals and of voluntary agencies concerned with the treatment and welfare of children with mental health problems. Support includes consultation and training and requires ready accessibility of the specialist services.

Service should be patient centred

There is inevitably a tension between accessibility and specialist services. When a child's problems cannot be adequately dealt with in primary care, specialist mental health professionals should be readily available. CAMHS require limited use of complex, hospital-based diagnostic facilities: most assessments and treatments can be adequately carried out in clinic or outpatient premises. When it is geographically desirable, the professional member of the solo professional or multi-disciplinary group should work on a sessional basis to cover more than one site. This will improve convenience for patients and relatives and enhance compliance with treatment. It is undesirable for families to travel long distances with disturbed children. Facilities should be convenient and appropriate for children and adolescents.

However if individual professionals work across several sites much time will be wasted in travel and there will be difficulty in forging good working links with other professional colleagues.

There should be patient choice

Wherever possible patients and carers should be informed about treatment possibilities and given a choice of the professions and services from which they would like advice and help.

Specialist services should accommodate the spectrum of need

Not all children and young people with mental health needs require multi-disciplinary resources. There should therefore be a solo professional service provided by child and adolescent psychiatrists, clinical psychologists specializing in work with children and young people, or child psychiatric nurses. This type of care facilitates the geographical spread of provision, whether organized as a uniprofessional service or as solo professionals doing outreach work from a multi-disciplinary base.

Multi-disciplinary resources should include psychiatrists, psychologists, psychotherapists, nurses and social workers, in order to provide for children and families with more complex needs. Speech and language and occupational therapists, and specialist teachers can make a contribution to such resources.

Where there are both unidisciplinary and multi-disciplinary groups, they should work in close liaison with each other and with social services and education colleagues to facilitate joint assessment and treatment. Multi-disciplinary resources may work as a team receiving referrals or as independent professional groups who collaborate on individual cases. Where a team organization is used professionals can also work in a solo or unidisciplinary mode. Team organization is needed for day and inpatient services. Inpatient services require educational provision.

Services should be concentrated in areas of greatest need

The prevalence of mental health problems in children and young people is high among those with special educational needs, those with developmental problems and physical illness, those with mental and physically ill parents and those in contact with social services and the law. Efforts should be made to ensure that services are distributed to provide maximum resource at points of greatest need.

Professional isolation should be avoided

It is unsatisfactory for professionals of any discipline to work in isolation. This can lead to undue work stress and idiosyncratic practice, as well as problems with the organization and continuity of service delivery. All services should therefore include at least two members of each professional group, one of whom should be of senior status.

Service organization

Services should have at least one senior member of each profession to organize and be responsible for intra-professional matters e.g. training, supervision, recruitment and service development. There should be clear management structures with lines of accountability for provision of services, incorporated by appropriate contracts or job plans.

Professional accountability

Professional accountability should be to an individual within the same discipline. There will need to be clear distinctions between the spheres of professional (clinical) and management responsibility.

Service isolation should be avoided

Solo professionals should have ready access to multi-disciplinary services, if staff are not also members of such services. There should be agreed procedures to prevent duplication of referrals to different services and mechanisms to distribute resources effectively and appropriately.

Good communication and collaboration are essential

If communication and collaboration are poor, resources will be wasted through duplication, there will be gaps in services and patients and carers will be confused.

Services can only be effective if there are easy and open channels of communication between all parties, independent of their management structure. This does not imply the need for a single management structure, but emphasizes the importance of a co-ordinating structure with shared strategies and policies.

The model of care

Localities

Each will have a primary care team, with a measure of specialist support from, for example, a school nurse or consultant community paediatrician who may work with several teams. Outreach services from child mental health professionals should be available in primary care as part of the solo professional specialist service.

Communities up to 250 000

Each should have both a solo professional and multi-disciplinary specialist service providing day and outpatient services. They should work closely with co-terminous local authority social services and education teams, preferably with some social workers and/or educational psychologists working from the same base. The model of co-ordination of solo and multi-disciplinary service can vary. What is essential is that the two components are co-ordinated. Two main models exist at the present time.

- Professionals collaborating in a multi-disciplinary service that also provides a solo service.
- Multi-disciplinary and solo professional services that are organizationally distinct but have mechanisms to collaborate effectively. In these circumstances the solo professional is usually a clinical psychology service.

The services will also work closely with the general paediatric and adult psychiatry services at the district general hospital. The specialist services will provide clinics at several sites, with the aim of ensuring that under-fives can be assessed reasonably close to their homes and that distance is not a barrier to care for older children. Intensive day treatment provision should be available for families of under-fives for parenting problems and for school age children. Day units need a range of dedicated staff similar to those in inpatient units. Local services for adolescents can be more concentrated, since this age group is likely to be more mobile and may be encouraged to attend by the availability of an environment which is sensitive to their interests and attitudes. Temporal as well as geographical access is important for this group: services should be available out of school hours. This also helps to ensure the attendance of parents who are working outside the home.

The specialist services should provide concentrated input in areas of high need, such as special schools, local authority family centres and residential homes and paediatric clinics. Joint approaches to funding of staff should be considered.

There should be access to hospital diagnostic facilities and inpatient paediatric beds on an occasional basis.

Communities of 750 000–1 000 000

Inpatient facilities for children and adolescents should be provided. An inpatient unit for younger children may be satisfactorily sited within a district general hospital, preferably close to outpatient and paediatric facilities. Adolescent units are best sited away from the district general hospital: access to investigatory, paediatric and adult mental health services is essential.

The Royal College of Psychiatrists has estimated that for a total population of 250 000 the inpatient provision should be 2–4 beds for children and 4–6 beds for adolescents up to the age of 16 in wards of a minimal size of 15 and 20–25 beds respectively.[205]

The inpatient facilities should be staffed by a dedicated, multi-disciplinary team which works closely with the community-based specialist services that will normally be the source of referrals. The inpatient team should include the following professional groups, as a minimum:

- child and adolescent psychiatrists
- clinical psychologists
- nurses
- occupational therapists
- social workers
- psychotherapists.

All inpatient units must have proper educational facilities (staffed by the local authority education department) and adequate recreational opportunities.

Adjacent outpatient and day care facilities can be helpful in managing the transition from inpatient to community-based care and eventual discharge.

Communities of 3 000 000

There are some rare and difficult-to-manage conditions for which highly specialist services are required. They can be divided into the following.

- Conditions needing complex assessment. For example:
  a) pervasive developmental disorders
  b) neuropsychiatric problems
  c) gender identity problems
  d) severe psychoses
  e) severe obsessional disorders
  f) complex child abuse
  g) sensory handicaps.
- Difficult treatment problems. For example:
  a) severe conduct disorders, including those needing secure accommodation
  b) other severe disorders not responsive to more local inpatient treatment (e.g. obsessional and mood disorders)
  c) neuropsychiatric disorders
  d) post-traumatic disorders
  e) severe epilepsy
  f) other brain dysfunction
  g) complex child abuse, including treatment of Münchausen Syndrome by Proxy and child/adolescent perpetrators of sexual abuse.

'Regional' centres are needed for these patients. These units are by definition dealing with highly demanding patients. It is essential that their staffing is maintained at a sufficiently high level to promote effective treatment and to prevent stress among staff.

Service targets

In a co-ordinated service for a population of 250 000 no professional should work in isolation. This means that both solo and multi-disciplinary services should have at least two professionals from any discipline, whether child psychiatry, clinical child psychology or community psychiatric nursing.

The targets for individual disciplines outlined below derive from recommendations from professional bodies where such recommendations exist. These recommendations do not take adequate account of the need for solo professional activity. Child psychiatrists and clinical psychologists will be expected to take a leading role in the development of solo and multi-disciplinary outpatient/day patient services, assessment, treatment, teaching and research. The involvement of senior nursing staff is vital for the planning of inpatient and most day patient services.

Psychiatrists

The Royal College of Psychiatrists recommends that there be 1.3 whole time equivalent (wte) consultants in child and adolescent psychiatry per 100 000 total population (for uni- and multi-disciplinary care). In addition to this there should be consultant provision for regional or supra-district services. In centres with a major teaching responsibility, consultant numbers should be increased to take account of teaching and research responsibilities.[205] Bridges over Troubled Waters has recommended that there should be 0.8 wte consultants per 200 000 population with a special responsibility for adolescent mental health services.[206] Child psychiatrists will usually be based in multi-disciplinary groups although some of their activity will be as a solo professional. All inpatient units need a child psychiatrist who carries appropriate responsibility for leadership and organization in collaboration with senior nursing staff.

Clinical psychologists

The Division of Clinical Psychology of the British Psychological Society recommends that there should be at least one full-time clinical psychologist working with children and families per 75 000 population. A child clinical psychologist at Grade B level with relevant skills and experience should head the psychology services for a given population. There should be at least one child clinical psychologist in all major service segments (e.g. under-fives, adolescents) provided by the unit or hospital trust. In a population of 250 000 a minimum of 3.5 wte posts are required. Additional posts will also be needed to provide specific services to specialist units for children and young people in primary health care.

Solo professional activity (page 22) is often appropriately conducted by clinical psychologists. This solo professional activity may be provided by clinical psychologists working from a multi-disciplinary base or a uniprofessional service.

Nurses

Nurses will usually be based within a multi-disciplinary group or team. They make an essential contribution to inpatient services but require additional training to work in an outpatient service. There are no specific recommendations for the expected levels of staffing for nurses working with multi-disciplinary outpatient groups. It is suggested that there should be a minimum of two community child psychiatric nurses for every consultant child psychiatrist. A day unit working intensively with between 50 and 80 children and their families per annum will require at least three full-time nursing staff of whom one should be at least Grade H. Inpatient units should maintain safe levels of staffing with trained nurses at all times. This may require a nurse: patient ratio of 1 : 1, depending on organizational arrangements in the unit.

Child psychotherapy

Psychotherapists perform a valuable role in both direct work with children and parents and in supporting and supervising intensive individual and group psychotherapy by other professionals. One child psychotherapist is required per 100 000 population with an additional child psychotherapist for every inpatient unit. The Child Psychotherapy Trust has proposed a target of one child psychotherapist for every child mental health team (a total of 660) with additional senior child psychotherapists who can take teaching responsibility.

Occupational therapy

Occupational therapists with specific training and expertise in working with children contribute towards day and inpatient treatment services. A minimum of one occupational therapist is needed per 100 000 population to work in day unit facilities. An additional occupational therapist will be required for every inpatient unit.

Social workers, educational psychologists and specialist teachers

Many children referred to child and adolescent mental health services are involved with social services or have special educational needs. Closely co-ordinated work is required in matters relating to child care, child abuse and educational difficulty. Ideally there should be three whole-time social workers per 100 000 population doing regular joint work with child and adolescent mental health services. There need to be arrangements to co-ordinate assessment and joint work with the school psychological service (educational psychologists). This is sometimes facilitated by co-location of educational psychologists with child and adolescent mental health services. As many children attending these services have specific educational difficulties, there can be significant benefit if some teachers with relevant specialist skills are co-located with the child and adolescent mental health services.

Support staff

Secretarial/administrative support staff are required: a ratio of one per three wte health professionals has been suggested, but this depends on organizational arrangements and office systems.

Range of services

The following range of non-residential services should be available in each district.

Assessment

- child and adolescent psychiatric, including neuro-psychiatric
- psychological including psychometry
- physical
- developmental
- educational
- social, including child protection.

Specific treatments

- cognitive and behavioural therapy
- individual child psychotherapy, including play therapy and art psychotherapy
- family therapy
- parental counselling, including marital therapy and advice on child management
- physical methods of treatment, including drug treatment
- social skills training
- special educational treatment
- day unit services
- consultation.

Group therapies should also be available (e.g. for social skills training or in the treatment of sexual abuse of child perpetrators of sexual abuse).

In addition resources should be available throughout the services for training (including continuing education).

Research

Service-related research is necessary to promote and monitor service developments and sustain the quality of staff activity. Appropriate resources are required.

Physical facilities

Within any district there should be at least one hospital and one community base for specialist child mental health professionals. The hospital base should be within a district general hospital or general teaching hospital, situated to enable satisfactory collaboration with paediatric and adult mental health and A and E services. All services should work in collaboration with community health services. Hospital and community clinic premises need to be dedicated and have:

- furnishing and equipment congenial for children and families
- toys and play equipment
- rooms suitable for the full range of assessments and treatments including physical examination, psychometry, individual psychotherapy, family therapy. Video facilities should be available
- an appropriate reception and waiting area
- clinic premises sympathetic to local culture to promote accessibility
- services for adolescents geared to their sub-culture with easy, direct access.

Contracts for care

Each commissioning authority will wish to ensure access for its population to the following.

- **Locally based specialist CAMHS** Provide regular, accessible solo and multi-professional assessment and treatment services, in liaison with other relevant professional groups. These are the 'core' services.
- **Inpatient units** Clear admission and discharge policies are needed and work in close co-operation with the local community-based specialist team is also needed. Commissioners should consider setting standards for waiting lists for admission to these units.
- **Specialist inpatient units for rare conditions** The patients requiring these services are often 'difficult-to-place' and their care is expensive. Purchasing authorities should decide how such cases will be dealt with and arrangements should be explicit in contracts. This may be done by requiring providers to deal with the matter, or by retaining contingency funds for such cases or by agreements on risk-sharing between purchasers and providers. In all cases a time limit for resolution of difficulties and appropriate placement of the child should be set. Clear arrangements also need to be agreed with local authorities about mechanisms for resolving problems relating to responsibility for care, with explicit systems for ensuring that children and families are not passed from one agency to another with unacceptable delays and deficiencies in care.

9 Outcome measures

Introduction

The general aim of child and adolescent mental health services is to relieve suffering in children with mental health problems, to support their families and promote their development into stable adults who fulfil their potential.

The assessment of outcome for specific problems can address:

- symptomatology
- general development
- impact on others
- long-term personal functioning.

It is nevertheless valuable to consider interim measures of structure and process as well as clinical outcomes.

Structure

Although the level of investment in a service is not in itself a measure of quality, it is clear that a seriously under-resourced service will not be able to provide acceptable care. Commissioners should bear in mind the manpower standards outlined in section 8 when specifying service requirements.

- Each commissioner should ensure that community-based specialist services are available to appropriate population groups (see section 8) and that there are clear systems of access to the service and from the service to inpatient and other specialist units when required.

- Specialist services should be set up in such a way that there are no isolated professionals.
- Services should have appropriate administrative and secretarial support to ensure efficient service provision.
- The level of provision should reflect local needs and take account of factors such as social disadvantage.
- Staffing and facilities should take account of local ethnic diversity.
- All premises should be appropriately equipped and furnished for the service age group (children or adolescents) to maximize acceptability and attendance.
- There should be a realistic quality standards framework and systems for service monitoring.

Process

Accessibility

- Clinics should be held at times which are convenient to school-age children and working parents.
- Clinics should be located in places accessible to parents of young children and individuals with disabilities.
- Clinics should be organized so that referrals are seen promptly for assessment, while the individuals are still motivated.
- Clinics should be organized so that there is minimal delay between assessment and the start of a treatment programme.
- Child and adolescent mental health staff should have regular, mutually agreed meetings with paediatric staff and there should be an on-call service for paediatric inpatients requiring urgent assessment (e.g. deliberate self-harm, abuse, psychosis).
- Specialist advice should be readily available to paediatricians, local authority social services, adult mental health, education and primary care services.

Communications

Explicit arrangements should be established for communications between the following.

- **Specialist professional staff** Especially for the multi-disciplinary assessment and monitoring of patients and co-ordination between solo and multi-disciplinary services.
- **Specialist professional staff and other health professionals** All those with responsibility for the health and welfare of children and adolescents with mental health problems and their families should be kept informed of treatment initiation, programmes and progress, subject where necessary to the normal constraints of confidentiality.
- **Services and clients** All those requiring treatment or support should be given a clear explanation of the nature of the problem, as assessed by specialist services, be informed about possible choices of management and be encouraged to participate actively in treatment. Where possible and in particular where this does not prejudice the welfare of the child assessment reports should be available to parents and care-givers.

Professional standards

The maintenance of professional standards of practice is an important, if indirect, consideration in ensuring satisfactory outcomes of care.

Purchasers should require that:

- all professional staff are qualified and registered with the appropriate body
- all professional staff have access to the time and resources needed for continuing education and professional development. There should be particular attention to training and treatment procedures where effectiveness has been demonstrated
- all professional staff participate in clinical audit, which is reported to the district or trust audit committee in accordance with local arrangements. An example of multi-disciplinary audit has recently been described[207]
- professional training taking place in the service is monitored by the appropriate professional body
- opportunities are available for research.

Outcomes

Clinical

Symptomatic

Some specific conditions allow direct measurement of outcomes. For example:

- specific phobias – proportion of those treated who overcome phobia
- enuresis – proportion of those treated who remain 'dry' for a specific time
- school refusal and truancy – proportion of children attending school regularly
- eating disorders – proportion of those treated who maintain a target weight and normal eating habits.

Goal attainment

In many cases progress cannot be assessed by symptomatic improvement and is measured by attainment of diverse treatment goals which are specific for each patient and include qualitative indicators. These goals should be identified for each referral and monitored at specified intervals. They should take into account the goals of parents, referrers and professionals and should be operationally defined.

Quality of life

The impact of treatment on the child and others can also be assessed by measures such as:

- school progress
- friendships
- family discord
- evidence of repeated abuse
- enjoyment of activity.

In all cases objective measures should be used. The C-GAS has been used in a number of services as a measure of impairment and its reduction.[208]

Adverse events

There are some adverse events which, though from time to time unavoidable, may require specific investigation through a confidential enquiry. This ensures that there were no service failures and allows procedures to be improved where necessary. These include:

- suicides under the age of 18 (whether or not under the care of mental health professionals)
- death or serious self-harm while under the care of child mental health services
- abuse while under the care of child mental health services
- pregnancy under the age of 16.

There are many other events or circumstances which may give rise to significant concern and could be used as a monitoring tool e.g. running away from home.

The clinical outcome of the treatment of child mental health problems may only become clear in later life. In many instances it is never known whether an apparently mildly successful intervention in reality prevented serious deterioration.

User satisfaction

The views of service users are an important aspect of outcome assessment. If users are unhappy with the service, they are likely to discontinue treatment and hence will not be able to benefit. It is particularly difficult to assess the satisfaction of users of child and adolescent mental health services since the designated patient may not be in a position to give an opinion and the interests and satisfaction of the carer or parent may not be concordant with those of the child. However many services have carried out evaluations of both client and referrer satisfaction. Purchasers should, however, encourage providers to develop approaches to this subject and report regularly on findings.

10 Targets

Introduction

Purchasers should aim for the provision of services and staff as set out in section 8. This would include:

- an adequately staffed solo professional and multi-disciplinary service for each 250 000 population
- geographically and temporally convenient services
- appropriate child-centred accommodation that facilitates the full range of assessment and treatment
- ready access to more specialist services, on a larger population base
- no isolated professional staff.

Specific targets

Specific service targets might include:

- no child or young person should wait more than four weeks after referral for specialist assessment by a local solo professional or multi-disciplinary team (a multi-disciplinary assessment is not necessary for every case)
- no child or young person should wait more than two weeks for the start of a treatment programme, following assessment
- a child who might require inpatient care should be assessed within 24 hours if the referring professional considers the case urgent
- a child who following assessment is considered in need of urgent inpatient care should be admitted within 24 hours
- a child requiring inpatient care that is not urgent should be admitted at an appropriate time, as advised by the clinician responsible for the case, and the family should be given at least one week's notice
- no child or young person should be admitted to an adult psychiatric inpatient unit unless there is a positive indication. If this is not considered an appropriate setting, the child or young person should be transferred to appropriate accommodation within one week
- in 'difficult-to-place' cases, senior staff in the authorities concerned (usually health and social services) should meet and decide which agency will take responsibility and set a timetable for placing the child in appropriate care
- all children or young people admitted to hospital or seen in A and E departments as a result of actual or suspected physical, sexual or emotional abuse should be referred for assessment. Local child protection procedures should clearly explain the correct mechanism. Social services will normally be the first line of assessment
- all children or young people admitted to hospital or seen in A and E departments as a result of deliberate self-harm should be seen by a child and adolescent psychiatrist before discharge or by a professional with appropriate training and ready access to a psychiatrist
- all provider units should have explicit procedures, copies of which are available to purchasers, for the two situations set out above.

11 Information

Introduction

Though there is considerable epidemiological information on child and adolescent mental health, clinical and management information is inadequate at present, although some services have produced local needs based assessments.[209] The situation is, of course, common to many other health services. It is particularly difficult in this service, however, because of the complex nature of some of the problems, the dependence of many of the designated patients on carers or other adults for referral to services, for participation in treatment and the multi-sectoral range of services. Information availability is variable and commissioners should check with professionals and other agencies on their local situation.

Areas for improvement

In order to improve needs assessment for child and adolescent mental health services, better information is needed on the following.

- **Mental health status in the community** This may require the development of instruments or other measures which can be realistically used in particular populations, though several standardized instruments are already available and screening for major disorders is possible.
- **Information on the number and location of high risk groups** These include relatively easy-to-identify groups, such as those in special schools, those in local authority care, or those with serious physical illness. It is also necessary however, to obtain better information on 'hidden' groups – poor achievers at school, children recently bereaved, children suffering following family break-ups, so as to intervene, if necessary, at an early stage and try to prevent the development of possible serious sequelae.
- **Information on the relationships between mental health and various environmental, social and economic factors** These may be useful proxies for health care needs (section 12).
- **Information from other providers** For example voluntary agencies.

Child and adolescent mental health services are essentially interdisciplinary: they involve different levels of health care and different agencies. Information should ideally be available to all professionals involved in care and integrated records of service use and care should be developed. Advances in information technology should enable more sophisticated systems to be used which could meet operational needs as well as service planning, research and monitoring requirements.

A coding framework such as the 'proposed core data set for child and adolescent mental health services' provides one example of the core data requirements for services.[15] In the medium term the read codes are likely to form the basis of an integrated health record of patient characteristics and core events, which will also cover child and adolescent mental health. At present there are very few operational systems that meet the full spectrum of information needs for these services.

12 Research priorities

Introduction

Child and adolescent mental health services share with most other clinical specialties serious omissions in knowledge about the effectiveness of interventions and the optimal organization of care. It is indeed to the credit of the specialty that so much has been achieved in areas fraught with methodological problems which are not encountered in, for example, surgical specialties with relatively clear cut outcome measures and a short time frame. The evidence available at present is sufficient to support purchasing decisions but there are important areas where further research would be valuable. Both the Medical Research Council and the Royal College of Psychiatrists have made recommendations for research priorities which have been taken into account in the development of these proposals.[210,211]

Research infrastructure

It is vital that appropriate staff and facilities are available within each population of 750 000 if there is to be satisfactory assessment of local needs and evaluated development of treatment and services. Both the Royal College of Psychiatrists and the British Psychological Society require trainees to undertake research. It is difficult for this to be achieved satisfactorily unless senior staff in academic departments engaged in research are available to provide support.

Normal and abnormal development

Research in this field is inevitably long term. Retrospective studies can produce useful and valid data. However prospective and follow-up studies are likely to be more reliable since they are not dependent upon retrospective recall but use information that has been collected for the purpose. The following areas of enquiry would merit further investigation.

Links between child and adult mental disorders

Which developmental characteristics and which mental problems in childhood predispose to which adult disorders? What is the strength and nature of the relationship? How do risk and protective factors during development influence outcome?[212]

The development of personality disorders in adolescence needs to be better understood.

Cross-generational influences

How do childrens' experiences of parent care at different stages of development affect their present mental health and subsequent psychological and emotional development?[213] It is particularly important to understand the influence of the contemporary changing patterns of family life and child care on child and adolescent mental health.

Genetic influences: interaction between genetic and environmental influences

Genetic influences on development and behaviour are increasingly recognized. The interaction between these and environmental influences need to be better understood. Certain conditions are particularly appropriate for genetic research. These include autism, learning difficulties and hyperkinetic disorders.

Differential response to environmental influences

Children within the same family vary in their mental health. Is this due to differences in individual resilience or vulnerability or in detailed family interactions? Can these be measured and does the evidence provide clues for prevention?[211]

Influence of brain dysfunction on mental health, including the interaction between brain function and environment

This is of particular importance for understanding the influence of different types of brain dysfunction on mental health. Increased collaboration between neuropsychiatry, paediatric neurology and child neuropsychology is required in studies of the psychological, social and educational consequences and management of neurological disorders and acquired dysfunction. Biological studies, including brain imaging, are likely to be of particular value.

Socio-economic relationships

The role of socio–economic factors in the genesis and maintenance of mental health problems is unclear. Research should examine the factors and mechanisms which determine why some children survive in conditions of psychosocial adversity while others do not.

Organization and standards of clinical practice

Development and evaluation of treatments

More research is needed across the range of treatments on effectiveness, with particular emphasis on longer term outcomes and the management of specific problems, including management in primary care.[212,213]

Development and evaluation of services

Studies are particularly needed of the relative merits of different service delivery settings (primary care, special care, special clinic, school) as well as modes of service delivery (direct intervention versus parent training and responsiveness to the needs of different communities and ethnic groups). Studies to improve recognition of mental health problems such as depression in primary care are needed.[213]

Developmental evaluation of preventive interventions

Examples of such research could include the prevention of conduct disorders and of psychiatric disorders in children with mental handicap.[213]

Developmental evaluation of specific treatments/interventions

Examples will include treatments for depression and difficulties arising from development characterized by Asperger's Syndrome and drug treatments.

Skill mix

What is the balance of uni– and multi–disciplinary service delivery? What are the costs and benefits of specific service delivery by different professional groups: to what extent is substitution feasible and desirable? Which problems are appropriately dealt with by voluntary agencies or primary health care?

Development of outcome measures

Since the ultimate outcome of child and adolescent mental health services is the child's success as an adult, valid interim measures need to be established. These should include clinical and quality of life measures.

Specific studies of special groups

Evidence on the effectiveness of care of specific groups of children and young people needs to be co-ordinated through broadly based research studies.

Examples are:

- 'hard-to-place' adolescents
- children in social services care
- children who have been abused[213]
- children and adolescents with challenging and/or persistent self-injurious behaviour
- childhood hyperactivity.[213]

Epidemiological studies

There would be particular value in local epidemiological studies to clarify service priorities by evaluating need for the different types of care. Some basic epidemiological work remains to be done.[212] In particular detailed studies are needed of those conditions which are, according to current evidence, increasing in incidence. These include:

- anorexia nervosa
- suicide
- juvenile delinquency
- depression.

Research in the field of child and adolescent mental health should normally be conducted by multi-disciplinary and multi-sectoral groups.

Attention also needs to be paid to the development and dissemination of research findings across the very broad range of professionals involved in the care of children. Research into this field, and the determinants of change in clinical practice would benefit both child and adolescent mental health services and other clinical specialties.

Priorities

Each of these areas for research is important for a number of reasons. There needs to be an overall balance between the more theoretical and academic studies and health services research. Both are needed to inform each other. However in terms of personal and social consequences, the aetiology, development and persistence of conduct disorders as well as their management and treatment in service settings should be given high priority.

Appendix I Definition of terms

- The term **care** is used to cover treatment, rehabilitation, counselling and social welfare.
- The term **service** covers **service agents** (formal and informal carers) and the **service settings**, varying from the domestic home to secure units.
- A **need** for care exists when an individual has an illness or impairment for which there is an effective and acceptable intervention. In this context an 'effective' intervention is one which achieves the treatment objective. It does not necessarily imply 'cure'. There will usually be a hierarchy of methods, from those which produce a complete and rapid recovery with no side-effects to those which achieve amelioration and/or secondary or tertiary prevention.

  The fact that needs are defined does not mean that they will be met. Some may remain unmet because other problems must be dealt with first, or because the more effective method is not available locally or availability is limited by rationing, or because the person in need or the carer objects. There are also 'potential' needs for forms of care that do not at the moment exist but which research may eventually provide.
- A **demand** for care exists when the individuals consider that they have a need and wish to receive care.
- **Utilization** occurs when an individual actually receives care.

  Need may not be expressed as demand; demand may not be followed by utilization; there can be demand and/or utilization without any need.
- **Professional** is a term used to encompass individuals such as GPs, nurses, health visitors, paediatricians, teachers and social workers who have a recognized professional qualification.
- **Specialist** is a term used to describe someone who has had specific training to work with individuals who have mental health needs. Child psychiatrists, clinical psychologists, psychiatric nurses, child psychotherapists and some social workers and teachers are the main groups with such specialist knowledge and skills.

Appendix II Core data set for child and adolescent psychology and psychiatric services

This list includes both problems and risk factors.

Anti-social (FA)
1. Tantrums/outbursts
2. Non-compliance at home
3. Stealing from home
4. Stealing other
5. Aggressive behaviour
6. Cruelty/violent brutality
7. Firesetting/destruction of property
8. Bullying/fighting
9. Substance abuse
10. Running away/wandering
11. Lying

School (FB)
1. School refusal/phobia
2. School non-attendance – other
3. School discipline problem

Cognition/abilities (FC)
1. Gifted
2. General learning disability
3. General academic under-achievement
4. Specific reading difficulty
5. Specific number difficulty
6. Specific spelling difficulty
7. Writing difficulty
8. Unusual cognitive pattern
9. Memory problems
10. Attention abnormality
11. Poor self-care skills

Self (FD)
1. Self-deprecation
2. Self-aggrandizement
3. Disability/disfigurement awareness

Mood (FE)
1. Irritability/moodiness
2. Fatigue/lassitude
3. Depression/misery
4. Euphoria/expansive disinhibition
5. Mood swings

Anxiety-related (FF)
1. General anxiety
2. Phobias
3. Separation anxiety

Self-regulation (FG)
1. Tics/habits/stereotypes
2. Obsessions/rituals
3. Overactivity
4. Enuresis/wetting
5. Soiling/constipation
6. Sleep/wake pattern problems
7. Problems during sleep
8. Subjective insomnia
9. Feeding problems/fads
10. Anorexia
11. Bulimia
12. Obesity/overeating

Social/relationships (FH)
1. Relationship difficulty parent/s/carers
2. Relationship difficulty other adults
3. Relationship difficulty siblings
4. General family relationships problems
5. Relationship difficulty peers
6. Harassment/persecution victim
7. 'Attention seeking' behaviour
8. Social disinhibition
9. Social withdrawal
10. Social sensitivity

Context (FI)
1. Marital difficulties
2. Family mental health problems
3. Family physical health problems
4. Adverse social circumstances

Life event (FJ)
1. Bereavement/loss
2. Stress reaction/adjustment reaction
3. PTSD/at risk for
4. Emergency/crisis during episode

Abuse/neglect (FK)
1. Failure to thrive
2. Neglect
3. Physical abuse
4. Emotional abuse
5. Sexual abuse

Self-harm/injury (FL)
1. Self-harm/overdose
2. Self-injurious behaviour
3. Risk-taking

Sexual and sex related (FM)
1. Inappropriately sexualized behaviour
2. Sexual misdemeanour/offence
3. Promiscuity/prostitution
4. Unusual/excessive solitary sexual activity
5. Concern about sexuality
6. Gender identity problem
7. Pregnancy

Personality/temperament (FN)
1. Shyness/social isolation
2. Personality/temperament extreme
3. Inappropriate immature behaviour

Speech and language (FO)
1. Mutism
2. Speech delay/disorder
3. Language delay/disorder

Autistic type characteristics (FP)
1. Autism/autistic features

Psychosis type characteristics (FQ)
1. Confusion/disorientation
2. Psychotic symptoms
3. Unusual/bizarre behaviour

'Psychosomatic' (FR)
1. Hypochondriasis
2. Factitious illness
3. Hysteria/conversion
4. Pain/discomfort non-organic origin
5. Headache

Physical illness/general paediatric (FS)
1. Non-neurological physical illness
2. Pain organic origin
3. Physical disability/deformity
4. HIV/AIDS
5. Other deteriorating organic condition
6. Terminal illness
7. Anxiety about physical medical procedures
8. Poor compliance with medical management

Physical/neurological (FT)
1. Physical slowness
2. Clumsiness/co-ordination difficulty
3. Epilepsy/turns/fits
4. Head injury

Sensory (FU)
1. Visual impairment
2. Blind
3. Hearing difficulties
4. Deaf

Genetic condition (FV)
1. Chromosome anomaly
2. Dysmorphic features
3. Behavioural phenotype

Normal limits (FW)
1. Parental concern but no clinical abnormality
2. Referrer concern but no clinical abnormality

Local other (FX)
1. *n* (Clinical problems locally specified)

Clinical features residual (FZ)
1. Other
2. Not known
3. Not coded

Appendix III Official statistics

Local data sources

Demographic

Basic demographic data covering the age and sex breakdown of a district population can be obtained from either the Public Health Common Data Set or the 1991 Census. These can be used to calculate the numbers within the 0–16 age group and to estimate the potential numbers of children with mental health problems. However the age bands used in the Common Data Set do not fully match those required to cover the 0–16 year olds as it uses the bands 0–4, 5–15 and 15–24 years. The Census, on the other hand, will allow analysis for single years of age. The Census also provides data on residence at ward level.

Ethnic

Both the Common Data Set and the Census provide data on the ethnic composition of district health authorities. The Common Data Set provides the percentage of heads of households born in the New Commonwealth or Pakistan. The 1991 Census provides data on the proportions of different minority groups within a district. The census also provides data on ethnic group by age categories (0–4, 5–15, 16–29).

Mortality

Deaths as a result of mental disorders classified under the ICD 9 codes for mental illness and suicide are classified by age and sex as part of a district's VS3 mortality statistics from OPCS.

Morbidity

Morbidity data can be obtained from a variety of sources. Hospital activity data on parasuicide and ICD codes for mental disorders can be obtained from the regional information system (RIS) or other relevant hospital administration systems (e.g. PAS). Hospital activity data provide a record of existing hospital service provision using the ICD codes for diagnosis. From this data it is possible to identify the age, admission method, postcode of patient, length of stay, etc. This data source will not include patients who are treated outside a district health authority area and will include patients from other districts who are treated in the provider unit. The RIS data will need to be interrogated by district code and data from the Mersey tapes (data on patients treated outside the relevant district health authority) added to this.

Hospital admission rates are as much a reflection of bed availability, referral rates and admission procedures as an indicator of need, but they can provide a useful guide on how need is currently being met. Hospital admission data also require care with interpretation as it is likely that an individual patient will be admitted more than once in a year and the data available are by admission episode and not by individual patient. This can result in an over-counting of some cases.

Some provider units have good data on attenders of psychiatric services as outpatients, inpatients or day care patients. The availability of data is not uniform or compulsory, however.

As an indicator of potential morbidity in the area of mental illness, disability and long-standing illness can be of relevance. Some health authorities and some local authorities keep a handicap register which holds details of children with either mental or physical disabilities. These are not compulsory and their completeness varies from place to place.

The Common Data Set contains details of selected congenital malformations; however, this only covers those malformations identified at or shortly after birth.

Details of limiting long-term illness can be obtained from the 1991 Census. The relevant age bands are 0–15 and 16–29. These data are divided into those resident in communal establishments and those resident in households.

Numbers of children with special educational needs and learning disabilities can be obtained from local education authorities. The Education Act of 1981 requires that children with special educational needs are statemented and their special need documented. This provides a source of information on intellectual and physical disability in an area but can be incomplete. Where a local education authority runs special schools, the number of children attending will be relatively easy to obtain.

Family and socio-economic data

Social class, unemployment rate, numbers receiving housing benefit, car ownership level, proportion of homes with basic amenities and housing tenure type can all indicate levels of social deprivation.

Details of housing tenure, dwelling type, access to cars, overcrowding and economic position can be obtained at ward level from the 1991 Census. Composite deprivation scores include the Jarman index and Townsend, both of which are available at ward level. The Common Data Set provides an underprivileged area score based on the 1981 Census; this may be of limited value because the data from the 1981 Census is now out of date. Local town councils can provide regular data on unemployment figures at ward level.

Criminality

Information on levels of crime among young people may be obtained from local police and probation services; however, this would involve requests in writing detailing exactly what data are required and permission will need to be obtained from the Chief Constable. However soft information can often be obtained informally by discussions with officers from these services.

Secondary data – based on national, regional and local authority areas

The following list provides a number of sources of data that provide a background picture of need and may be of value in determining service requirements for child and adolescent mental health.

Ethnic

Details of the percentage population in each ethnic group for 1983, 1989, 1990 and 1991 – *GHS 1991*, OPCS. Available from public or academic libraries.

Detailed information about the ethnic data provided by the 1991 Census and information on the use of the Labour Force Survey to estimate Britain's ethnic minority population – *Population Trends No. 72*, Summer 1993, pp. 12–17, OPCS. Available from public and academic libraries.

Hospital activity

Admissions to NHS hospitals for mental illness and mental handicap by age group (under ten, 10–14, 15–19) for 1978–1990 including age-specific rates per 100 000 population – *Health and Personal Social Statistics for England*, 1992 edition, HMSO. Tables 9.2 and 9.4. Available from public and academic libraries.

Morbidity

Physical illness – percentages of children reported as having long-standing illness by age bands (0–4, 5–15) – *Regional Trends No. 27*, 1992, p. 69, Table 6.3. Available from public and academic libraries.

Self-reported sickness by age (0–4, 5–15) and sex and economic status for 1972–91. Percentage reporting: **a** long-standing illness; **b** limiting long-standing illness; **c** restricted activity in last 14 days. *GHS 1991*, Tables 8.1–8.4. Available from public and academic libraries.

Social services information

Children and young people on child protection register 1993 – *DoH Personal Social Services (A/ F92/ 13)*. Data on children included in child protection registers for different regions of England by abuse category. Available from public and academic libraries, or from: The Statistician, SD3A Room 454, Skipton House, 80 London Road, Elephant and Castle, London SE1 6LW.

Children accommodated in secure units 1993 – *DoH Personal Social Statistics (A/ F92/ 21)*. Data on children accommodated in secure units both within and outside child's care authority, lists of secure units, etc. Available from public and academic libraries, or from: The Statistician, SD3A Room 454, Skipton House, 80 London Road, Elephant and Castle, London SE1 6LW.

Children in care in local authorities 1993 – *DoH Personal Social Statistics (A/ F91/ 12)*. Information on the numbers of children in each different region of England, reasons for admission to care, etc. Available from public and academic libraries, or from: The Statistician, SD3A Room 454, Skipton House, 80 London Road, Elephant and Castle, London SE1 6LW.

Socio-economic information

Usual gross weekly household income by family type for married couples, lone mothers and lone fathers – *GHS 1991*, Table 2.30, p. 28. Unemployment rates by socio-economic group and sex, Tables 5.7 and 5.8. Available from public and academic libraries.

Unemployment

Percentage of unemployed by age and sex for 1992 – Table 7.15. Unemployment rates for years 1981–91 for regional areas of England – Table 7.16, and households by economic status of head for 1991 – Table 7.5. *Regional Trends No. 27*, 1992. Available from public and academic libraries.

One parent families – trends in the number of one parent families in Great Britain – *Population Trends No. 71*, Spring 1993. Demographic characteristics of one parent families in Great Britain – *Population Trends No. 65*, Autumn 1991.

Children in families broken by divorce – *Population Trends No. 61*, Autumn 1990. Available from public and academic libraries.

Details of the number of dependent children by family type and marital status of lone mothers – *GHS 1991*, Table 2.20. Available from public and academic libraries.

Criminality

Young offenders found guilty or cautioned by type of offence and age (10–13, 14–16, 17–20) in 1981 and 1991 – data covers different regions of England – *Regional Trends No. 28*, 1993, Table 9.6. Available from public and academic libraries.

Supervision orders and intermediate treatment year ending March 1991. *DoH Personal Social Statistics (A/F9/16)*. Available from: The Statistician, SD3A Room 454, Skipton House, 80 London Road, Elephant and Castle, London SE1 6LW.

Appendix IV Current service status for child and adolescent mental health services

Much of the following information has been derived from a recent survey of services for the mental health of children and young people in the UK.[149] It looks at purchasing authorities and the various aspects of child and adolescent services, including community-based care, inpatient and special units, day treatment services, clinical psychology services, paediatric services, social services, education and the non-voluntary sector.

Purchasing authorities

69 of 121 (57%) purchasing authorities were included in the survey. 52% (36 authorities) had done developmental work on a specific strategy for mental health services for young people and 28% (19) had such a strategy in use. A third had consulted with at least four departments or agencies in developing this strategy. The remaining 33 authorities (48%) reported that they had no specific strategy.

In 62% (43) of authorities included in the study, the current specification was separate from that of adult mental health services. Only nine (13%) purchasing authorities had a basis for their specification that was related to the needs of their population i.e. either a formal needs assessment or at least three other indicators of need.

In 55% (38) of authorities, the current contract was separate from that of adult mental health services. In a fifth of cases a single contract was in place covering community, day and inpatient care for children and for adolescents. Every purchasing authority had contracts with named provider units for inpatient care, or else mentioned that they used extra-contractual referrals (8%), or either a block regional contract or a subscription system (7%).

In 28% of authorities, older adolescents (aged 16 to 18 years) were included in the same contract as younger age groups; in 16% they were included by design in the contracts for adult mental health; in 17% they were included with adults, by default.

In most cases the work of clinical psychologists was included within wider contracts, but separate contracts with clinical psychology were specified by 7% of authorities. In 13% of authorities the main contract included services to be provided in education and/or social services.

Plans for evaluation of the service were largely undeveloped.

Child and adolescent mental health services

The specialist child and adolescent mental health services are largely delivered from a community base, by means of multi-disciplinary teams. Within these teams psychiatrists and social workers are almost universal members, although the number of social workers has reduced in the past three years, mainly as a result of local authority reorganization. Numbers of staff and the range of skills available vary widely between different units. There is little regular input to the service from the education sector.

Community-based care

Of the 151 (81%) departments of child and adolescent mental health included in the survey, 94% provided a service in community clinics; 19% were an integral part of units also providing inpatient care and also 11% provided care on a day basis. 70% provided a community service only. There was a designated budget for child and adolescent psychiatry in 56% of services.

There is major variation in the distribution of numbers of child and adolescent psychiatrists across the country and in the type of work they undertake. 15% of services had less than one wte consultant, 40% between one and two, and 44% more than two. The number of children (aged 0–18 years) per one wte consultant ranged from 6 403 to 244 135. The number of wte consultants per 100 000 child population ranged from 0.41 to 15.62. Child and adolescent psychiatrists provided emergency cover in 69% of districts.

Other professional staff included:

- 58% had junior medical staff in training positions
- 69% had clinical psychologists
- 44% had a psychotherapist
- 17% had a family therapist
- 11% had an educational psychologist
- 63% had a psychiatric community nurse
- 81% had a social worker.

Provision to other professional groups included:

- 36% of departments provided five or more sessions (half-day duration) per month to paediatrics. 27% provided no services to paediatrics
- 11% provided sessions in general practice (majority were one session per week)
- 35% provided more than five regular sessions a month for social services departments
- 28% provided five or more regular sessions a month to schools
- 18% provided occasional sessions for the police and 8% for the probation service
- 37% did sessions for voluntary sector agencies.

Overall 15% provided no, or very limited, services to any other department.

Inpatient and special units

Many inpatient units, including former regional adolescent units, are experiencing problems particularly with respect to the new system of contracting for services.

Of the 37 NHS inpatient units (60%) who replied, 32% had contracts with a single purchasing authority, 22% with two authorities and 41% had multiple contracts.

Staffing revealed:

- consultants – 8% of units had less than one wte while 51% had two or more
- 95% had junior medical staff
- 76% had clinical psychology input
- 65% had an occupational therapist
- all but one had teachers
- 32% of units had psychotherapy
- 70% of units had social work input.

65% had a distinct and separate budget, but only 23% held it themselves within child and adolescent psychiatry.

25% of units catered for both children and adolescents, a further 25% for children only and 50% for adolescents only.

60% functioned on a seven-day basis, while 40% closed at the weekend. 80% provided 24-hour cover for emergencies.

33% provided care entirely in one location.

Innovative or specialist clinics and other services most frequently mentioned included child sexual abuse/post-abuse therapy, parenting and early intervention, eating disorders, early onset psychoses, severe enuresis, communication disorders/neuropsychiatry and autism.

Day treatment services

A quarter of all units (37) replied that they provided treatment on a day basis. Of these 59% also provided inpatient care.

Of these units:

- 95% had at least one wte consultant
- 89% had junior medical staff
- 78% had a clinical psychologist
- 84% had a social worker
- the median number of psychiatric community nurses was four.

33% of units stated that treatment on a day basis was available somewhere within the district. A further 10% used education authority facilities, such as emotional and behavioural difficulty (EBD) units or social services day centres as a base from which to provide day treatment. Facilities in neighbouring districts were often otherwise available.

Clinical psychology services

Clinical psychology is a growing profession, working increasingly from an independent base. Clinical psychologists still work mainly with child and adolescent mental health teams, but they also provide direct and consultative services to acute and community services in other sectors of the NHS, to social services and to other agencies.

Of the 168 (90%, covering 88% of districts) clinical psychology services who replied, 67% provided some care on a unidisciplinary basis and 25% had separate contracts with GP fundholders.

The responses covered 513 clinical psychologists, comprising 156 grade B and 357 grade A. There were 277 trainees and 18% of responses stated that their work was essential to maintain the present level of service. In 13% of services other professional staff were employed, including counsellors.

In the past three years, 44% of the services had seen no change in the numbers of clinical psychologists; in 36% there had been an increase and in 12% a reduction. 30% reported that an increase was planned for next year.

42% received referrals from child and family or child guidance clinics. Many clinical psychologists worked regular sessions with acute paediatrics, on the wards (36% of services) and in outpatients (46%). Sessions were provided as required by 27% in cases of deliberate self-harm and by 29% in cases of emergency admissions for abuse. Even more (61%) did sessions in child development clinics and in 20% of services this amounted to more than 20 sessions a month (the equivalent of a half-time post).

The third most important area of work was for social services, with regular commitment from 57% of clinical psychology departments.

Only 8% of services gave more than the occasional sessions in mainstream schools, but 18% provided regular sessions in special schools for children with learning difficulties, physical disabilities or sensory impairment.

On a smaller scale, sessions were provided for the police and probation services by 10% of services, largely on an occasional basis. Similarly 10% of services provided a small input to drug and alcohol services. 32% worked with the voluntary sector, helping particularly with training and management.

22% of clinical psychology departments were members of a multi-disciplinary group that gave advice to the purchasing authority.

Paediatric services

Data from this survey suggest that more children with emotional and behavioural disorder present to paediatricians than to any other profession. Paediatric training in the main does not prepare them for this and they would welcome further opportunities to gain relevant experience.

Hospital paediatrics

It is estimated that 5–15% of children referred to paediatric departments is due primarily to emotional and behavioural problems. The main conditions were: constipation/encopresis/soiling (54% of directorates), enuresis (42%), headaches/abdominal pain/psychosomatic conditions (34%), sleep problems (34%) and feeding problems (27%).

Paediatricians estimated that 15% (median) of their patients had an underlying or additional emotional or behavioural disorder in addition to the main presenting condition, although 42% of departments suggested a lower proportion (between 3% and 10%).

29% of hospital-based paediatric consultants felt that their training had adequately prepared them for dealing with emotional and behavioural problems, although 46% stated that training was still inadequate in this respect. Junior staff needed regular placements or an opportunity to participate in clinics in child and adolescent psychiatry.

Psychological training and support for nurses and junior doctors was regularly provided in 37% of departments. 70% of departments said they needed more support and training for staff in these types of problem.

48% of paediatric departments held formal planning sessions together with the child and adolescent psychiatry department; 32% were part of a multi-agency group, advising the purchasing authority on children's needs, including those for mental health services.

Community paediatrics

20% of children referred to community paediatricians were referred primarily for emotional and behavioural problems. The main sources of referral were health visitors (reported by 83% of departments), GPs (64%) and educational authority staff such as teachers and educational psychologists (53%).

22% of community paediatricians said that they referred between 40% and 50% of cases for further opinion. The main emotional and behavioural conditions treated were largely the same as those treated by hospital paediatricians.

Community paediatricians, even more so than hospital paediatricians, felt that the resources for child and adolescent psychiatry in their district were quite inadequate. Long waiting lists and frequent personnel changes were described by 75%.

Community paediatricians were involved formally in planning provision with the child and adolescent psychiatry teams in 56% of districts. They were represented on a multi-agency group advising the purchasing authority for these services in 40%.

Social services

Social services departments concentrate resources on children in need, many of whom have serious emotional and behavioural problems. They report unsatisfactory access to NHS specialist expertise in children's mental health.

Social service departments contribute to mental health services by providing social work input to the multi-disciplinary team in 81% of services. Of the 59 (56% covering 62% of health authorities) social services departments who replied, 17% had no formal or written policy on assessment and therapeutic services for children and young people with emotional and behavioural problems. All others had some sort of policy, though often part of a general policy for children in need, based on the Children Act. 46% were either working on, or had already developed, joint policies or joint commissioning with the health service. A further 9% had firm plans to start negotiations in this particular field with the NHS in the coming year. Five departments had also included the local education authority in policy making.

Assessment and therapeutic services for children and young people were mostly provided in social services family or day centres (in 29% of departments), though in 17% child guidance centres were used. 20% negotiated provision of part of the service by the NHS; a very small number stated that they purchased these services.

49% of social services departments were represented on a multi-agency group to advise the NHS purchaser. A large proportion (75%) had representation on a multi-agency group to plan services with the NHS providers.

61% of respondents stated that they had had no staff losses in the last three years and 56% said they had had staff increases during that time. Other changes that might have had an effect on services for this client group included the establishment of new team structures (mentioned by 20%) and this was frequently linked with the need to meet the requirements of the Children Act.

64% of the departments stated that they ran services or programmes specifically for children with emotional and behavioural difficulties, providing group, family and individual sessions. The social services department had a direct input into schools in 54% of authorities. 86% of departments contributed on a regular or occasional basis to health services, with half providing sessions in at least five different health settings. The most common contribution was to child and family (psychiatric) outpatient or community-based clinics (58% of the responses), followed quite closely by work in child development clinics (51%), paediatric inpatient wards (49%) and children's outpatient clinics (42%).

Work with the police and the probation service was carried out by a number of authorities, although 30% did not do anything in this respect.

61% of social services departments had direct input into voluntary or joint SSD/voluntary facilities. 12% stated that they had firm plans to increase work with the voluntary sector in the coming year.

The education sector

Local education authorities are greatly concerned with emotional and behavioural difficulties in their pupils. Behaviour support services, as currently provided in three-quarters of local education authorities, include assessment of the educational needs of pupils with severe behaviour problems, but frequently no relevant medical contribution is included. Special schools for children with emotional and behavioural difficulties report that few pupils have statements in which therapeutic help is specified, although the head teachers consider that nearly half of all pupils would benefit from such help.

Local education authorities

Of the 29 (27%) local education authorities who replied, 59% had developed a policy for pupils in mainstream education who had, or were at risk of, emotional and behavioural problems. A further 17% were currently reviewing their policy.

Educational psychology services

Of the 47 (44% covering 45% of health districts) educational psychology services who replied, work in this field was specifically included in the job descriptions of 55% of services.

Special schools for children with emotional and behavioural problems

Of the 165 (approximately 55%) special schools who replied, 80% felt that help from the referring agency was token in that children were rarely visited by specialists from home and that the resources available from the referring agencies were inadequate. Similarly 86% did not feel that the NHS provided resources that the children needed.

90% of schools had provided in-service training for teaching staff on emotional and behavioural problems or related issues in the past year.

Non-teaching specialists with a particular role in therapeutic support were not widely or regularly available.

64% of EBD schools had not been visited by child and adolescent psychiatrists in the past year. 36% had been, 68% of them on a regular basis.

The non-statutory sector

The voluntary sector plays a large part at primary care level, particularly in providing services such as counselling, and taking many self-referrals. Voluntary organizations also act as a filter to specialist mental health and social services. Since the NHS mental health services accept self-referrals less and less, the voluntary services may be filling a gap in provision. They offer particular expertise for secondary and tertiary provision.

15% of the child and adolescent psychiatry services stated that they had used private hospitals for inpatients. Several responses mentioned that the major and sole use was for eating disorders, such as anorexia nervosa.

In planning (including health needs assessment), 42% of NHS purchasing authorities said that they had included voluntary organizations in their discussions and several had involved particular organizations in a substantial way.

A detailed study of data for one region (Yorkshire) revealed 154 independent or semi-independent organizations, covering all cities and towns in the region. 42% were classified as providing a service for a range of general problems that were of concern to young people. 18% provided services to help people misusing drugs, alcohol or other substances. 12% provided services for children and young people who had been abused sexually, physically or emotionally. About 8% of organizations helped children or their families with problems related to serious physical illness or disability. Another 8% specialized in problems surrounding homelessness.

25% specifically provided for the 16 to 25 age group and 14% for the under 16s.

The sources of funding were varied and few relied entirely on one source. 51% received some local authority funding, including grants from social services, education and housing departments. 6% specifically mentioned joint funding from health and social services. 8% received some funding from central government. 46% raised at least part of their costs by general fundraising, through appeals, corporate fundraising, grants from trusts and subscriptions. 6% charged for their services, either directly or through contracts.

Psychiatric community nurses

There were 260 wte nurses working in community-based units, of whom 47% had been specifically trained in children's and adolescent's psychiatric care (ENB 603). Of the 87 units who employed a community psychiatric nurse (CPN) only one-third (34%) had a nurse with this qualification. Of nurses working within inpatient units less than one-fifth (18%) had undertaken the ENB course, though there were only four units with no nurse with this qualification.

Child psychotherapy

Child psychotherapists working in community-based units were unevenly distributed across the country with 92% employed in the four Thames regions, Wessex, Oxford and South Western.

References

1 Rutter M. Pathways from childhood to adult life. *J Child Psychol Psych* 1989; **30**: 23–51.

2 Garmezy N, Rutter M. Acute reactions to stress. In *Child and Adolescent Psychiatry: Modern Approaches* (eds M Rutter and L Herzov). Oxford: Blackwell Scientific Publications, 1985, pp. 152–76.

3 Rutter M, Cox A. Other family influences. In *Child and Adolescent Psychiatry: Modern Approaches* (eds M Rutter and L Herzov). Oxford: Blackwell Scientific Publications, 1985, pp. 58–81.

4 Wolkind S, Rutter M. Separation, loss and family relationships. In *Child and Adolescent Psychiatry: Modern Approaches* (eds M Rutter and L Herzov). Oxford: Blackwell Scientific Publications, 1985, pp. 34–57.

5 Shaw D, Emery R. Chronic family adversity and school age children's adjustment. *J Am Ac Child Adol Psych* 1988; **27**: 200–6.

6 Goodyer I. Family relationships, life events and child psychopathology. *J Child Psychol Psych* 1990; **31**: 161–92.

7 Goodyer I. Life events and psychiatric disorder. *J Child Psych Psych* 1990; **31**: 839–48.

8 Farrington DP, Loeber RG, van Kammen WB. Long-term criminal outcomes of hyperactivity-impulsivity-attention deficit and conduct in childhood. In *Straight and Devious Pathways from Childhood to Adulthood* (eds LN Robins and M Rutter). Cambridge: Cambridge University Press, 1990, pp. 62–81.

9 Harrington R. *Depression disorder in childhood and adolescence*. Chichester: Wiley, 1993.

10 Brown GW, Harris TO, Bifulco A. Long-term effects of early loss of parent. In *Depression in young people: developmental and clinical perspectives* (eds M Rutter, CE Izard, PB Read). New York: Guilford Press, 1985, pp. 251–96.

11 Rutter M (ed.). *Studies of Psychosocial Risk*. Cambridge: Cambridge University Press, 1988.

12 Brewin CR, Wing JK. *The MRC Needs for Care Assessment Manual*. London: Institute of Psychiatry, 1988.

13 Mathew GK. Measuring need and evaluating services. In *Problems and progress in medical care* (ed. G McLachlan). Sixth series. Oxford: Oxford University Press, 1971.

14 Wing JK, Brewin C, Thornicroft G. Defining mental health needs. In *Measuring Mental Health Needs* (eds G Thornicroft, C Brewin, Wing JK). London: HMSO, 1993, chapter 1.

15 Berger M, Hill P, Sein E *et al. A proposed core data set for child and adolescent psychology and psychiatry services.* Association for Child Psychology and Psychiatry, 1993.

16 World Health Organization. *International Statistical Classification of Diseases and Related Health Problems.* Tenth Revision. Geneva: WHO, 1992.

17 Rutter M, Smith DJ. *Psychological Disorders in Young People. Time trends and their causes.* Chichester: Wiley, 1995.

18 Cox AD. Preventive aspects of child psychiatry. *Arch Dis Child* 1993; **68**: 691–701.

19 Graham PJ. Prevention. In *Child and Adolescent Psychiatry: Modern Perspectives* (eds M Rutter, E Taylor, L Hersov). 3rd edn. Oxford: Blackwell Scientific Publications, 1994, pp. 815–28.

20 Department for Education. *Pupils with Problems: Circulars 8–13/94.* London: Department for Education, 1994.

21 Department of Health. *Child Protection: Message from Research.* London: HMSO, 1995.

22 Richman N, Stevenson JE, Graham PJ. Prevalence of behaviour problems in 3 year old children: an epidemiological study in a London borough. *J Child Psych Psych* 1975; **16**: 277.

23 Rutter M, Cox A, Tupling C *et al.* Attainment and adjustment in two geographical areas. I: The prevalence of psychiatric disorder. *Brit J Psych* 1975; **126**: 493.

24 Rutter M, Graham P. The reliability and validity of the psychiatric assessment of the child. *Brit J Psych* 1968; **114**: 563.

25 Verhulst FC, Berden GFG, Sanders-Woudstra JAR. Mental health in Dutch children. II. *Act Psych Scan* 1985; **72**: 1.

26 Costello EJ. Developments in child psychiatric epidemiology. *J Am Ac Child Adol Pysch* 1988; **28**: 836.

27 Graham P, Rutter M. Psychiatric disorder in the young and adolescent. *J Roy Soc Med* 1973; **66**: 1226–9.

28 Rutter M, Graham P, Chadwick O *et al.* Adolescent turmoil: fact or fiction? *J Child Psychol Pysch* 1976; **17**: 35–56.

29 Offor DR, Boyle MH, Szatmari P *et al.* Ontario Child Health Study. II. Six month prevalence of disorder and rates of service utilisation. *Arch Gen Psych* 1987; **44**: 832.

30 Rutter M, Yule W, Berger M *et al.* Children of West Indian immigrants. 1. Rates of behavioural deviance and psychiatric disorder. *J Child Psychol Psych* 1974; **15**: 241–62.

31 Cochrane R. Psychological and behavioural disturbance in West Indians, Indians and Pakistanis in Britain. A comparison of rates among children and adults. *Brit J Psych* 1979; **134**: 201.

32 Hackett L, Hackett R, Taylor DC. Psychological disturbance and its association in the children of the Gujarati community. *J Child Psychol Psych* 1991; **32**: 851–6.

33 Rack P. Psychiatric disorder in immigrants. In *Readings in Psychiatry 3*. Oxford: Medical Education Sevices, 1984, pp. 53–7.

34 Rack P. *Race, culture and mental disorder.* London: Tavistock, 1982.

35 Kallarackal AM, Herbert M. The happiness of Indian immigrant children. *New Soc* 1976; **35**: 422.

36 Hackett L, Hackett R. Parental ideas of normal and deviant child behaviour. A comparison of two ethnic groups. *Brit J Psych* 1993; **162**: 353–7.

37 Rutter M, Yule W, Graham P. Enuresis and Behavioural Deviance: some epidemiological considerations. In *Bladder Control and Enuresis* (eds I Kolvin, R MacKeith, SR Meadow). Clinics in Developmental Medicine, nos 48/49. London: Heinemann/Spastics International Medical Publications, 1973.

38 Jarvelin MR, Vikevainen-Tervonen L, Moilanen I *et al.* Enuresis in seven year old children. *Acta Paed Scand* 1988; **77**: 148–53.

39 Minde K, Minde R. *Infant psychiatry: an introductory text.* London: Sage Publications, 1986.

40 Apley J, Nalsh N. Recurrent abdominal pains: a field study of 1000 children. *Arch Dis Child* 1958; **33**: 165–70.

41 Apley J. *The Child with Abdominal Pains.* 2nd edn. Oxford: Blackwell Scientific Publications, 1975.

42 Zahner GEP, Clubb MM, Leckman JF *et al.* The epidemiology of Tourette's Syndrome. In *Tourette's Syndrome and Tic Disorders* (eds DJ Cohen, RD Bruun, JF Leckmann). New York: Wiley, 1988, p.79.

43 Rutter M, Tizard J, Whitmore K. *Education, Health and Behaviour.* London: Longmann, 1970.

44 Berger M, Yule W, Rutter M. Attainment and adjustment in two geographical areas II: the prevalence of specific reading retardation. *Brit J Psych* 1975; **126**: 510-19.

45 Benjamin RS, Costello EJ, Warren M. Anxiety disorders in a paediatric sample. *J Anx Dis* 1990; **4**: 293–316.

46 Kashani JH, Orvaschel H. Anxiety disorders in mid-adolescence: a community sample. *Am J Psychiatry* 1988; **145**: 960–4.

47 Offord DR, Boyle MH, Jones BA. Psychiatric disorder and poor school performance among welfare children in Ontario. *Can J Psych* 1987; **32**: 518.

48 Offord DR, Boyle MH, Racine YH. *Ontario Child Health Study: Children at risk.* Toronto: Queen's Printer for Ontario, 1990.

49 Shapiro AK, Shapiro ES, Young JG *et al.* (eds) *Gilles de la Tourette Syndrome.* 2nd edn. New York: Raven, 1988.

50 Flament MF, Whitacker A, Rapoport J *et al.* Obsessive compulsive disorder in adolescence. *J Am Ac Child Adol Psych* 1988; **27**: 764–77.

51 Whitacker A, Johnson J, Shaffer D *et al.* Uncommon troubles in young people: prevalence estimates of selected psychiatric disorders in a non-referred adolescent population. *Arch Gen Psych* 1990; **47**: 487–96.

52 Taylor E, Sandburg S, Thorley G *et al.* *The Epidemiology of Childhood Hyperactivity. Maudsley Monographs no. 33.* Oxford: Oxford University Press, 1991.

53 Bellman M. Studies on encopresis. *Acta Paed Scand* 1966; suppl: 170.

54 Nielson S. The epidemiology of anorexia nervosa in Denmark from 1973 to 1987: a nationwide register study of psychiatric admission. *Acta Psych Scand* 1990; **81**: 507-14.

55 Steinhausen H-C, Seidal R. A prospective follow-up study in early-onset eating disorders. In *The Course of Eating Disorders: Long-Term Follow-Up Studies of Anorexia and Bulimia Nervosa Course* (eds W Herzog, HC Deter, W Vandereycken). Berlin: Springer, 1992.

56 Freidman JM, Asnis GM, Boeck M *et al.* Prevalence of specific suicidal behaviour in high school samples. *Am J Psych* 1987; **144**: 1203–6.

57 Smith K, Crawford S. Suicidal behaviours among 'normal' high school students. *Suicide Life Threat Behav* 1986; **16**: 313–25.

58 Pfeffer CR, Newcorn J, Kaplan G *et al.* Suicidal behaviour in adolescent psychiatric patients. *J Am Acad Child Adol Psych* 1988; **27**: 357–61.

59 Shaffer D, Fisher P. The epidemiology of suicide in children and young adolescents. *J Am Acad Child Psych* 1981; **20**: 545–65.

60 Shaffer D, Piacentini J. Suicide and Attempted Suicide. In *Child Psychiatry: Modern Approaches* (eds M Rutter, L Hersov, E Taylor). 3rd edn. Oxford: Blackwell Scientific Publications, 1994.

61 Office of Population Censuses and Surveys. *Adolescent Drinking.* London: HMSO, 1992.

62 Swadi H. Drug and Substance Use Among 3333 London Adolescents. *Brit J Add* 1988; **83**: 935–42.

63 Health Education Authority. *Tomorrow's Young Adults. 9–15 Year Olds Look at Alcohol, Drugs, Exercise and Smoking.* London: Health Education Authority, 1992.

64 Mott J. Self-reported cannabis use on Great Britain in 1981. *Brit J Add* 1985; **80**: 37–43.

65 Miller JD, Cisin IH, Gardenere-Keaton H *et al.* *National Survey on Drug Abuse: Main Findings. National Institute on Drug Abuse Research Monograph.* Rockville, MD: National Institute on Drug Abuse, 1983.

66 Johnson LD, O'Malley PM, Bachman JG. *Drug Use among American High School Students, College Students and other Young Adults: National Trends Through 1985. National Institute on Drug Abuse Research Monograph.* Rockville, MD: National Institute on Drug Abuse, 1986.

67 Coggans S, Davies J. *National Evaluation of Drug Education in Scotland: Final Report.* Strathclyde: University of Strathclyde, 1989.

68 Farrell M. Ecstasy and the oxygen of publicity. *Brit J Add* 1989; **84**: 943.

69 Ashton M. *Drug Misuse in Britain: National Audit of Drug Misuse Statistics.* London: ISDD, 1991.

70 Breslau N. Psychiatric disorder in children with disabilities. *J Am Acad Child Psych* 1985; **24**: 87.

71 Pless IB. Clinical assessment. Physical and psychological functioning. *Ped Clin North Am* 1984; **32**: 33.

72 Satter-White B. Impact of chronic illness on child and family. An over-view based on five surveys. *Int J Rehab Res* 1978; **1**: 7.

73 Cadman D, Boyle M, Szatmari P *et al.* Chronic illness, disability and mental and social well-being. Findings of the Ontario Child Health Study. *Paed* 1987; **79**: 805.

74 Rutter M. Brain damage syndrome in childhood. Concepts and findings. *J Child Psychol Psych* 1977; **18**: 1.

75 Goodman R. Brain disorders. In *Child Psychiatry: Modern Approaches* (eds M Rutter, L Hersov, E Taylor). 3rd edn. Oxford: Blackwell Scientific Publications, 1994.

76 Brown G, Chadwick O, Shaffer D *et al.* A prospective study of children with head injuries, III. Psychiatric sequalae. *Pyschol Med* 1981; **11**: 63.

77 Goodman R. Brain development. In *Development Through Life: A Handbook for Clinicians* (eds M Rutter, DF Hay). Oxford: Blackwell Scientific Publications, 1994.

78 Martin JAM. Aetiological factors relating childhood deafness in the European Community. *Audiol* 1982; **21**: 149–58.

79 Bamford J, Saunders E. *Hearing impairment, auditory perception and language disability*. 2nd edn. London: Whurr, 1991.

80 Rutter M, Graham P, Berger M. *A neuropsychiatric study in childhood. Clinics in Developmental Medicine. Nos 35/36*. London: Spastics International Medical Publications, 1970.

81 Fundulis T, Kolvin I, Garside RF. *Speech retarded and deaf children: Their Psychological Development*. London: Academic Press, 1979.

82 Schlesinger H, Meadow KP. *Sound and Sign*. Cambridge: University of California, 1972.

83 Hill AE, McKendrick P, Poole JJ *et al*. The Liverpool Visual Assessment Team: 10 Years Experience. *Child: Care, Hlth Develop* 1986; **12**: 37–51.

84 Felce D, Taylor D, Wright K. *People with learning difficulties. Project 12. Epidemiologically based needs assessment*. DHA Project: Research programme, 1992.

85 Graham PJ. Behavioural and Intellectual Development in Childhood Epidemiology. *Brit Med Bull* 1986; **42(2)**: 155–62.

86 West DJ, Farrington DP. *Who becomes delinquent?* London: Heinemann, 1973.

87 Hoy E, Weiss G, Minde K *et al*. The hyperactive child at adolescence: Cognitive, emotional and social functioning. *J Abnormal Child Psychol* 1978; **6**: 311.

88 Minde K, Lewin D, Weiss G *et al*. The hyperactive child in elementary school: A five-year controlled follow-up. *Exceptional Child* 1971; **38**: 215.

89 Emslie G, Rush AJ, Weinberg W *et al*. *Self-report of depressive symptoms in adolescents: Ethnic and sex differences*. Paper presented at the annual meeting of the American Academy of Child and Adolescent Psychiatry. Washington, DC, 1987.

90 Fleming JE, Offord DR, Boyle MH. Prevalence of childhood and adolescent depression in the community: Ontario Child Health Study. *Brit J Psych* 1989; **155**: 647.

91 Friedrich WN, Reams R, Jacobs JH. Sex differences in depression in early adolescents. *Psychol Reports* 1988; **62**: 475.

92 Garrison CZ, Schoenbach VJ, Kaplan BH. Depressive symptoms in early adolescence. In *Depression in multidisciplinary perspective*. New York: Brunner-Mazel, 1985, pp. 60–82.

93 Hoberman HM, Garfinkel BD, Parsons JH *et al*. Depression in a community sample of adolescents. Paper presented at the annual meeting of the American Academy of Child and Adolescent Psychiatry. Los Angeles, 1986.

94 Reynolds WM, Coats KI. Depression in adolescence: incidence, depth and correlates. Paper presented at the 10th International Association of Child and Adolescent Psychiatry and Allied Professions. Dublin, 1982.

95 Terr LC. The use of the Beck Depression Inventory with Adolescents. *J Abnormal Child Psychol* 1982; **10**: 277.

96 Costello EJ, Costello AJ, Edelbrock C *et al*. Psychiatric disorders in paediatric primary care. *Arch Gen Psych* 1988; **45**: 1107.

97 Williams S, McGee RO, Anderson J *et al*. The structure and correlates of self-reported symptoms in 11 year old children. *J Abnorm Child Psychol* 1989; **17**: 55.

98 Richman N, Stevenson JE, Graham PJ. *Pre-school to school: a behaviour study*. London and New York: Academic Press, 1982.

99 Baker L, Cantwell DP. Psychiatric disorder in children with different types of communication disorder. *J Commun Dis* 1982; **15**: 113–26.

100 Beitchman JH, Nair R, Clegg M *et al.* Prevalence of psychiatric disorders in children with speech and language disorders. *J Am Acad Child Adol Psych* 1986; **25**: 528–35.

101 Frick PJ. Family dysfunction and the disruptive behaviour disorders. In *Advances in Clinical and Child Psychology* (eds TH Ollendick, RJ Prinz). Vol. 16. New York: Plenum Press, 1994.

102 Farrington DP, West DJ. The Cambridge study in delinquent development (United Kingdom). In *Prospective Longitudinal Research: An empirical basis for the primary prevention of psychological disorders* (eds SA Mednick, AE Baert). Oxford: Oxford University Press, 1981, pp. 133–45.

103 Patterson GR. *Coercive Family Process.* Eugene, Oregon: Castalia Publishing Company, 1982.

104 Earls F, Yung KG. Temperament and home environment characteristics as causal factors in the early development of childhood psychopathology. *J Am Acad Child Adol Psych* 1987; **26**: 491.

105 Emery RE, O'Leary KD. Children's perceptions of marital discord and behavioural problems of boys and girls. *J Abnorm Child Psychol* 1982; **10**: 11.

106 Rutter M. Epidemiological-longitudinal strategies and causal research in child psychiatry. *J Am Acad Child Psych* 1981; **20**: 513.

107 Zill N. Divorce, marital conflict and children's mental health: Research findings and policy recommendations. Testimony before the Subcommittee on Family and Human Services, US Senate Committee on Labour and Human Resources Senate Hearing 98–195. Washington, DC: US Government Printing Office, 1983, pp. 90–106.

108 Monck E, Graham P, Richman N *et al.* Adolescent girls I: Background factors in anxiety and depressive states. *Brit J Psych* 1994; **165**: 760–9.

109 Monck E, Graham P, Richman N *et al.* Adolescent girls II: Background factors in anxiety and depressive states. *Brit J Psych* 1994; **165**: 770–80.

110 Office of Population Censuses and Surveys. *General Household Survey.* Series GHS. No. 22. London: HMSO, 1992.

111 Haskey J. Patterns of marriage, divorce and cohabitation in the different countries of Europe. *Europ Pop Trends* 1992; **69**: 27–36.

112 Kiernan K, Wickes M. *Family Change and Future Policy.* Family Policies Study Centre, 231 Baker Street, London NW1 6XE, 1990.

113 Jones MB, Offord DR, Abrams N. Brothers, sisters and anti-social behaviour. *Brit J Psych* 1980; **136**: 139.

114 Offord DR, Fleming JE. *Child and Adolescent Psychiatry. A Comprehensive Textbook* (ed. M Lewis). Baltimore: Williams and Wilkins, 1989.

115 Leckman JF, Weissman MM, Merikangas KR *et al.* Major depression and panic disorder. *Psychopharmacol Bull* 1985; **21**: 543.

116 Weissman MM, Merikangas KR, Gammon GD *et al.* Depression and anxiety disorders in parents and children. Results from the Yale Family Study. *Arch Gen Psych* 1984; **41**: 845.

117 Gottesman II, Shields J. *Schizophrenia: The Epigenic Puzzle.* Cambridge: Cambridge University Press, 1982.

118 Rutter M, Giller H. *Juvenile Delinquency: Trends and Perspectives.* New York: Penguin Books, 1983.

119 Robins LN, West PA, Herjanic BL. Arrests and delinquency in two generations: a study of black urban families and their children. *J Child Psychol Psych* 1975; **3**: 241.

120 Osborn SG, West DJ. Conviction records of fathers and sons compared. *Brit J Criminol* 1979; **19**: 120–33.

121 McCord W, McCord J. *Origins of Crime.* New York: Columbia University Press, 1959.

122 Rutter M. Family and school influences: meanings, mechanisms and implications. In *Longitudinal studies in child psychology and psychiatry* (ed. AR Nicol). Chichester: Wiley, 1985.

123 Dilalla LF, Gottesman I. Heterogeneity of causes for delinquency and criminality: life-span perspectives. *Develop Psychopathol* 1989; **1**: 339–49.

124 Brown K, Saqui S. Parent–child interaction in abusing families and its possible causes and consequences. In *Child Abuse: The Educational Perspective* (ed. P Maher). Oxford: Basil Blackwell, 1987.

125 Erickson MF, Egeland B, Pianta R. The effects of maltreatment on the development of young children (eds D Cicchetti, V Carlson). In *Child Maltreatment*. Cambridge: Cambridge University Press, 1989.

126 Finkelhor D. *A Sourcebook on Child Sexual Abuse*. Beverly Hills: Sage, 1986.

127 Kelly L, Regan L, Burton S. *An exploratory study of the prevalence of sexual abuse in a sample of 16–21 year olds*. London: University of London, 1991.

128 Earls F. Prevalence of behaviour problems in 3 year old children: a cross-sectional replication. *Arch Gen Psych*, 1980; **37**: 1153.

129 Achenbach TM, Edelbrook CS. Behavioural problems and competences by parents of normal and disturbed children aged four through to sixteen. *Monograph Society Res Child Develop* 1981; **46**: 1.

130 Lapouse R, Monk MA. Behaviour deviations in a representative sample of children: variation by sex, race, social class and family size. *Am J Orthopsych* 1964; **34**: 346.

131 Anderson J, Williams S, McGee R *et al*. Cognitive and social correlates of DSM-III disorders in preadolescent children. *J Am Acad Child Adol Psych* 1989; **28**: 842.

132 Offord DR. Social factors in the aetiology of childhood disorders. In *Handbook of studies on child psychiatry* (eds B Tonge, G Burrows, J Werry). Amsterdam: Elsevier, 1990, pp. 56–68.

133 Banks M, Jackson P. Unemployment and risk of minor psychiatric disorder in young people: cross-sectional and longitudinal evidence. *Psychol Med* 1982; **12**: 786–98.

134 Farrington DP, Gallagher B, Morley L *et al*. Unemployment, school leaving and crimes. *Brit J Criminol* 1986; **26**: 335–56.

135 Quinton D. Urbanisation and child mental health. *J Child Psychol Psych* 1988; **29**: 11–20.

136 Richman N. The effects of housing on pre-school children and their mothers. *Develop Med Child Neurol* 1974; **16**: 53–8.

137 Alperstein G, Arnstein E. Homeless children – a challenge for pediatricians. *Ped Clin North Am* 1988; **35**: 1413–25.

138 Fox SJ, Barrnett J, Davies M *et al*. Psychopathology and developmental delay in homeless children. *J Am Acad Child Adol Psych* 1990; **29**: 732–5.

139 Wolkind S, Rutter M. Socio-cultural factors. In *Child and Adolescent Psychiatry: Modern Approaches* (eds M Rutter, L Hersov). 2nd edn. Oxford: Blackwell Scientific Publications, 1985.

140 Olweus D. Bully/victim problems among school children: basic facts and effects of a school based intervention program. In *The Development and Treatment of Child Aggression*. Erlbaum, Hillsdale, New Jersey, 1991.

141 Pynoos RS, Frederick C, Nader K *et al*. Life threat and post-traumatic stress in school-age children. *Arch Gen Psych* 1987; **47**: 1057–63

142 Yule W. The effects of disasters in children. *Ass Child Psychol Psych News* 1989; **11**: 3–6.

143 Yule W. Children in shipping disasters. *J Roy Soc Med* 1991; **84**: 12–15.

144 Goodyer IM. Development psycholpathology: the impact of recurrent life events in anxious and depressed school age children. *J Roy Soc Med* 1994; **87**: 327–9.

145 Masterman SH, Reams R. Support groups for bereaved preschool and school-age children. *Am J Orthopsych* 1988; **58**: 562–70.

146 Birtchnell J. Early parent death and mental illness. *Brit J Psych* 1970; **116**: 281–8.

147 Brown GW, Harris T, Copeland JR. Depression and loss. *Brit J Psych* 1971; **130**: 1–18.

148 Black D. Annotation: The bereaved child. *J Child Psychol Psych* 1978; **19**: 287–92.

149 Kurtz Z, Thornes R, Wolkind S. *Services for the Mental Health of Children and Young People in England – A National Review*. London: Maudsley Hospital and South Thames (West) Regional Health Authority, 1994.

150 Stevenson J. Health visitor-based services for pre-school children with behaviour problems. Association for Child Psychology and Psychiatry. *Occasional papers No. 2*. London: ACPP, 1990.

151 Barker W, Anderson R. The Child Develoment Programme: an evaluation of process and outcomes. Evaluation Document 9. Manuscript. Early Child Development Unit. Bristol: University of Bristol, 1988.

152 Hughes T, Garralda ME, Tylee A. *Child Mental Health Problems: A Booklet on Child Psychiatry for General Practitioners*. London: St Mary's CAP, 1994.

153 Steinberg D, Yule W. Consultative work. In *Child and Adolescent Psychiatry: Modern Approaches* (eds M Rutter, L Hersov). 2nd edn. Oxford, Blackwell Scientific Publications, 1985, pp. 914–26.

154 Lask B. Paediatric liaison work. In *Child and Adolescent Psychiatry: Modern Approaches* (eds M Rutter, L Hersov, E Taylor). 3rd edn. Oxford: Blackwell Scientific Publications, 1994, pp. 996–1005.

155 Hibbs ED. Child and adolescent disorders: issues for psychological treatment research. *J Abnorm Child Psychol* 1995; **23**: 1–10.

156 Gadow KD. Pediatric psychopharmacotherapy: a review of recent research. *J Child Psychol Psych* 1992; **33**: 153–95.

157 Barnett RJ, Docherty JP, Frommelt GM. A review of child psychotherapy research since 1963. *J Am Acad Child Adol Psych* 1991; **30**: 1–14.

158 Pfeiffer SI, Strzelecki SC. Inpatient psychiatric treatment of children and adolescents: a review of outcome studies. *J Am Acad Child Adol Psych* 1990; **29**: 847–53.

159 Graziano AM, Diament DM. Parental behaviour training: an examination of the paradigm. *Behav Mod* 1992; **16**: 3–38.

160 Allen JS, Tarnowski KJ, Simonian SJ *et al.* The generalization map revisited: Assessment of generalized treatment effects in child and adolescent behavior therapy. *Behav Therap* 1991; **22**: 393–405.

161 Weisz JR, Weiss B. Assessing the effects of clinic-based psychotherapy with children and adolescents. *J Consult Clin Psychol* 1989; **57**: 741–6.

162 Weisz JR, Donenberg GR, Hann SS *et al.* Child and adolescent psychotherapy outcomes in experiments versus clinics: why the disparity? *J Abnorm Child Psychol* 1995; **23**: 83–106.

163 Kovacs M, Lohr WD. Research on psychotherapy with children and adolescents: an overview of evolving trends and current issues. *J Abnorm Child Psychol* 1995; **23**: 11–30.

164 March JS. Cognitive-behavioural psychotherapy for children and adolescents with OCD: a review and recommendations for treatment. *J Am Child Adol Psych* 1995; **34**: 7–16.

165 Earls F. Oppositional-defiant and conduct disorders. In *Child and Adolescent Psychiatry: Modern Approaches* (eds M Rutter, L Hersov, E Taylor). 3rd edn. Oxford: Blackwell Scientific Publications, 1994, pp. 308–29.

166 Campbell M, Adams PB, Small AM *et al.* Lithium in hospitalized aggressive children with conduct disorder: a double-blind trial and placebo-controlled study. *J Am Acad Child Adol Psych* 1995; **34**: 445.

167 Alessi N, Naylor MW, Ghaziuddin M *et al.* Update on lithium carbonate therapy in children and adolescents. *J Am Acad Child Adol Psych* 1994; **33**: 291–304.

168 Kazdin AE, Siegal TC, Bass D. Cognitive problem-solving skills training and parent management training in the treatment of anti-social behavior in children. *J Consult Clin Psychol* 1992; **60**: 733–47.

169 Kazdin AE. The effectiveness of psychotherapy with children and adults. *J Consult Clin Psychol* 1991; **59**: 785–98.

170 Offord DR, Bennett KJ. Conduct disorder: long-term outcomes and intervention effectiveness. *J Am Acad Child Adol Psych* 1994; **33**: 1069–78.

171 Ryan ND. The pharmacologic treatment of child and adolescent depression. *Psych Clinic North Am* 1992; **15**: 29–40.

172 Ambrosini PJ, Bianchi MD, Rabinovich H *et al*. Anti-depressant treatment in children and adolescents. I. Affective disorders. *J Am Acad Child Adol Psych* 1993; **32**: 1–6.

173 Ambrosini PJ, Bianchi MD, Rabinovitch H *et al*. Antidepressant treatments in children and adolescents. II. Anxiety, physical and behavioral disorders. *J Am Acad Child Adol Psych* 1993; **32**: 483–93.

174 Harrington R. Affective disorders. In *Child and Adolescent Psychiatry: Modern Approaches* (eds M Rutter, L Hersov, E Taylor). 3rd edn. Oxford: Blackwell Scientific Publications, 1994, pp. 330–50.

175 Reynolds WM. Depression in Adolescents: Contemporary Issues and Perspectives. In *Advances in Clinical and Child Psychiatry* (eds TH Ollendick, RJ Prinz). Vol. 16. New York: Plenum Press, 1994, pp. 261–316.

176 Coffey BJ. Anxiolytics for children and adolescents: traditional and new drugs. *J Child Adoles Psychopharmacol* 1990; **1**: 57–83.

177 Bernstein GA, Borchardt CM. Anxiety disorders of childhood and adolescence: a critical review. *J Am Acad Child Adol Psych* 1991; **30**: 519–32.

178 Dadds M, Heard PM, Rapee RM. Anxiety disorders in children. *Int Rev Psych* 1991; **3**: 231–41.

179 King N, Tong BJ. Treatment of childhood anxiety disorders using behaviour therapy and pharmacotherapy. *Austr NZ J Psych* 1992; **26**: 644–51.

180 Klein RG. Anxiety disorders. In *Child and Adolescent Psychiatry: Modern Approaches* (eds M Rutter, L Hersov, E Taylor). 3rd edn. Oxford: Blackwell Scientific Publications, 1994, pp. 351–74.

181 Steinhausen H. Anorexia and bulimia nervosa. In *Child and Adolescent Psychiatry: Modern Approaches* (eds M Rutter, L Hersov, E Taylor). 3rd edn. Oxford: Blackwell Scientific Publications, 1994, pp. 425 41.

182 Rapaport J, Swedo SH, Leonard H. Obsessive-compulsive disorders. In *Child and Adolescent Psychiatry* (eds M Rutter, L Hersov, E Taylor). 3rd edn. Oxford: Blackwell Scientific Publications, 1994, pp. 441–54.

183 Piacentini J, Jaffer M, Graae F. The psychopharmacologic treatment of child and adolescent obsessive compulsive disorder. *Psych Clin North Am* 1992; **15**: 87–107.

184 Taylor E. Syndromes of attentional deficit and hyperactivity. In *Child and Adolescent Psychiatry: Modern Approaches* (eds M Rutter, L Hersov, E Taylor). 3rd edn. Oxford: Blackwell Scientific Publications, 1994, pp. 285–307.

185 Jacobvitz D, Sroufe AL, Stewart M *et al*. Treatment of attentional and hyperactivity problems in children with sympathomimetic drugs: a comprehensive review. *J Am Acad Child Adol Psych* 1990; **29**: 677–88.

186 Greenhill LL. Pharmacologic treatment of attention deficit hyperactivity disorder. *Psych Clin North Am* 1992; **15**: 1–27.

187 DuPaul GJ, Barkley R. Behavioural contributions to pharmacotherapy: the utility of behavioural methodology in medication treatment of children with attention deficit hyperactivity disorder. *Behav Therap* 1993; **24**: 47–65.

188 Leckman JF, Cohen DJ. Tic disorders. In *Child and Adolescent Psychiatry: Modern Approaches* (eds M Rutter, L Hersov, E Taylor). 3rd edn. Oxford: Blackwell Scientific Publications, 1994, pp. 455–66.

189 Skuse D. Feeding and sleeping disorders. In *Child and Adolescent Psychiatry: Modern Approaches* (eds M Rutter, L Hersov, E Taylor). 3rd edn. Oxford: Blackwell Scientific Publications, 1994, pp. 467–89.

190 Zeanah CH, Emde RN. Attachment disorders in infancy and early childhood. In *Child and Adolescent Psychiatry: Modern Approaches* (eds M Rutter, L Hersov, E Taylor). 3rd edn. Oxford: Blackwell Scientific Publications, 1994, pp. 490–504.

191 Lord C, Rutter M. Autism and pervasive developmental disorders. In *Child and Adolescent Psychiatry: Modern Approaches* (eds M Rutter, L Hersov, E Taylor). 3rd edn. Oxford: Blackwell Scientific Publications, 1994, pp. 569–93.

192 Werry JS, Taylor E. Schizophrenic and allied disorders. In *Child and Adolescent Psychiatry: Modern Approaches* (eds M Rutter, L Hersov, E Taylor). 3rd edn. Oxford: Blackwell Scientific Publications, 1994, pp. 594–646.

193 Green R. Atypical psychosexual development. In *Child and Adolescent Psychiatry: Modern Approaches* (eds M Rutter, L Hersov, E Taylor). 3rd edn. Blackwell Scientific Publications, 1994, pp. 749–58

194 Mrazek DA. Psychiatric aspects of somatic disease and disorders. In *Child and Adolescent Psychiatry: Modern Approaches* (eds M Rutter, L Hersov, E Taylor). 3rd edn. Oxford: Blackwell Scientific Publications, 1994, pp. 697–710.

195 Skuse D, Bentovim A. Physical and emotional maltreatment. In *Child and Adolescent Psychiatry: Modern Approaches* (eds M Rutter, L Hersov, E Taylor). 3rd edn. Oxford: Blackwell Scientific Publications, 1994, pp. 209–29.

196 O'Donohue WT, Elliott AN. Treatment of the sexually abused child: a review. *J Clin Child Psychol* 1992; **21**: 218–28.

197 Jones DP. The untreatable family. *Child Abuse Neglect* 1987; **11**: 409–20.

198 Smith M, Bentovim A. Sexual abuse. In *Child and Adolescent Psychiatry: Modern Approaches* (eds M Rutter, L Hersov, E Taylor). 3rd edn. Oxford: Blackwell Scientific Publications, 1994, pp. 230–51.

199 Lorion RP, Myers TG, Bartels C *et al.* Preventive intervention research. In *Advances in Clinical and Child Psychology* (eds TH Ollendick, RJ Prinz). Vol. 16. New York, Plenum Press, 1994, pp. 19–39.

200 McMillan HL, McMillan JL, Offord DR *et al.* Primary prevention of child physical abuse and neglect: a critical review. Part I. *J Child Psychol Psych* 1994; **35**: 835–56.

201 McMillan HL, McMillan JL, Offord DR *et al.* Primary prevention of child sexual abuse: a critical review. Part II. *J Child Psychol Psych* 1994; **35**: 857–76.

202 Kolvin I, Garside RF, Nicol AR *et al. Help starts here: The Maladjusted Child in Ordinary School.* London, New York: Tavistock, 1981.

203 St Leger AS, Schneiden H, Walsworth-Bell JP. *Evaluating Health Service Effectiveness.* Milton Keynes: Open University Press, 1992.

204 Levitt EE. Psychotherapy with children: an evaluation. *J Consult Psychol* 1957; **21**: 189–96.

205 Royal College of Psychiatrists. *Mental Health of the Nation: the contribution of psychiatry: a report of the President's Working Group.* London: Royal College of Psychiatrists, 1992.

206 Health Advisory Service. *Bridges over Troubled Waters: A Report from the NHS Health Advisory Service on Services for the Disturbed Adolescents.* London: Department of Health, 1986.

207 Leahy A, Thambirajah MS, Winkley LM. Multidisciplinary audit in child and adolescent psychiatry. *Psych Bull* 1992; **16**: 214–5.

208 Shaffer D, Gould MS, Brasie J *et al.* Children's Global Assessment Scale. *Arch Gen Psych* 1983; **40**: 1228–31.

209 Light D, Bailey V. *A Needs-Based Purchasing Plan for Child Based Mental Health Services.* London: North West Thames Regional Health Authority, 1992.

210 Research Committee of the Royal College of Psychiatrists. Future directions for research in child and adolescent psychiatry. *Psych Bull* 1991; **15**: 308–10.

211 Medical Research Council. *Field Review of Biological Psychiatry.* London: Medical Research Council, 1993.

212 McGuffin P. *Mental Health: Priorities in Research for the 1990s.* London: Mental Health Foundation, 1989.

213 Department of Health. *Central Research and Development Committee: Mental Health Research and Developmental Priorities.* London: Department of Health, 1992.

Index